STOP FEEDING US LIES

How health and happiness come to those who seek the truth

CHARLIE SPEDDING

Published in Great Britain
2019 by CS Books
Spedding Partnership
Durham
www.stopfeedinguslies.com

A catalogue record for this book is available from the British Library.

Cover design by Emma Nicole Harker

ISBN 978-0-9563296-1-5

CONTENTS

Introduction

ACKNOWLEDGEMENTS

In my search for the truth, I have been inspired and informed by the works of many independently-minded people, without whom this book would not have been possible. Their names include: Prof. Tim Noakes, South Africa; Dr Gary Fettke, Australia; Dr Jason Fung, Canada; Dr Zoe Harcombe, Wales; Dr Malcolm Kendrick, Scotland; Dr Michael Eades, America; Dr Andreas Eenfeldt, Sweden; Allan Savory, Zimbabwe; Dr Frederic Leroy, Belgium; Dr Georgia Ede, America; Dr Robert Lustig, America; Ivor Cummins, Ireland; Nina Teicholz, America; and many others.

This book would not have been written without the unwavering support, and editing skills, of my wife Christina.

Introduction

My father was a Pharmacist. When I was a child, he referred to himself as a Dispensing Chemist and his business was a Chemist shop. Nowadays we would call it a Community Pharmacy. I was fascinated by all the jars and bottles of tablets and potions that filled the shelves of his dispensary and even more intrigued to hear about all the diseases these could treat. I decided that I wanted to work in such an interesting place, whilst helping people to be healthy. I followed in my father's footsteps and became a Pharmacist too.

I spent most of the next 35 years trying to improve people's health but I left the Pharmacy profession earlier than I had intended to, feeling greatly disillusioned. The majority of patients in a community setting (known as Primary Care) are suffering from metabolic diseases like high blood pressure or diabetes. People with severe and immediate health problems are in hospital or specialist units (Secondary Care). Most of the people I was seeing every day had problems that required medication but they were not in imminent danger. In recent years it struck me more and more that these patients never got better. They were taking medication that relieved some of their symptoms but didn't tackle the cause of their disease. Thousands of people were going to be taking drugs for the rest of their lives without ever being cured of their illness. This is a fantastic business model for the pharmaceutical industry but it is not why I became a Pharmacist, and I don't want to be one anymore.

The other thing I have done with my life is to run. I was a competitive athlete for 20 years. I joined Gateshead Harriers when I was 16, and 16 years later I won the London Marathon and a Bronze Medal in the Los Angeles Olympic marathon. This achievement was at the far end of my wildest dreams and had looked extremely unlikely for the first 12 years of my running career. During that time I followed a method of training that was generally regarded as the ideal programme for distance runners. It had been used by triple-Olympic Champion, Peter Snell, and other great runners under the tutelage of the New Zealand coach, Arthur Lydiard. During those 12 years I ran quite well but after suffering from many injuries and always feeling I could do better, I decided to change both my mental approach and my physical training. The next four years brought constant improvement and huge success. I had been told to follow the accepted doctrine of the time but it didn't work for me. When I rejected the conventional approach and did something different, I amazed myself, and many others, by how much I improved.

In 2012 I began to wonder if accepted wisdom about health was another example of dogma that wasn't as good as everyone thought. I have spent the last seven years researching this topic. As an athlete I had always believed in the importance of exercise for health and as a Pharmacist I had always believed in the importance of medicine. While these both have their place, I now believe that by far the most crucial element of living a healthy, happy life is the food we eat. I have discovered that the advice we are given by the health authorities is hopelessly wrong. The way we are told to eat is inadequate for some people and catastrophic for others. The global obesity crisis has occurred as a direct result of the official dietary guidelines. All those people in my pharmacy with metabolic diseases are never going to be cured by medicine but they could be healthy with the right food. We live in an era where the food industry feeds us with no thought for our health and the health industry treats us with no thought for our food. I have learnt so much since I left my medical career, I feel compelled to write this book and help people to be well, healthy and happy – at last.

Chapter 1

STOP ASKING THE WRONG QUESTION

What costs the UK £340 million every day but doesn't do what it is supposed to? The answer is the National Health Service. A health service for the nation ought to make the nation healthy but for the last 35 years we have all become increasingly ill. The number of people suffering from obesity, diabetes, cancer and mental disorders has risen continuously, along with the amount of money spent on dealing with all these problems. The money involved is extraordinary. The budget for the 2017/18 financial year is 124 billion pounds. The enormous cost of free health care has been increasing every year for the last seven decades. This system isn't working. If the NHS was truly successful, the cost of the service should be going down each year as people become well, but they are not well. More people are being treated but the population is not healthier. Clearly, there is something wrong.

The NHS is a much-loved institution and politicians from every party always support it. Even in times of austerity, they happily give more money to the health service whilst being forced to reduce the money that goes into so many other services. There is a constant debate about how much extra money the health service needs and political parties vie with each other to appear to be the most generous towards the cost of our healthcare services. The questions about the NHS seem to be endless. How much extra money should we spend? How many doctors and nurses do we need? How many hospitals should we have? How should services be organised? Should we have Family Health Authorities, or Primary Care Trusts or Local Commissioning Bodies? How should GPs be paid? Which services should they offer and which services should pharmacists and dentists be paid for? These questions are debated repeatedly and changes are implemented over and over again. But, however they organise it, the budget for the health service goes up every year; it never goes down. It seems clear to me that nobody is asking the right question. All these questions are important but ultimately futile unless you can answer the most important question of them all, which is, "Why are so many people ill?"

I believe we have been misled and misinformed for years. We have been told by experts and authorities how to be healthy, what to eat and what to do. I am going to show you why nearly all of this advice is wrong. We need to see through all the myths, misinformation and lies that we have been told for the past four decades. Throughout the course of this book, I am going to ask you to do something that is very difficult for the human mind to do. I am going to ask you to unlearn the things that you have always been told are true.

These are some of the well-known, often repeated statements, issued by the organisations giving us our official nutritional advice:

1. We should base our meals on starchy carbohydrates like bread, potatoes and pasta.
2. We should choose low-fat foods whenever we can.
3. We should minimise our intake of saturated fat.
4. We should use polyunsaturated vegetable oils instead of butter and lard.
5. We should minimise our intake of salt.
6. We should keep our cholesterol levels as low as possible.
7. When eating meat, we should only eat lean meat.
8. We should drink between two and four litres of water every day.
9. To lose weight, we should restrict our calorie intake.
10. To lose weight, we should take more exercise.

I suspect we are all familiar with each of these statements and many of us will have acted upon them. However, all of these declarations are wrong. These ideas have not made us healthy; they have caused obesity, diabetes, cancer and a wide range of mental disorders. I have searched for and found the proof that our dietary advice is nonsense. I have written this book to reveal the truth about health, happiness and weight loss.

Wretched lives and horrible deaths

I have always believed that an understanding of the past helps us not only to put our present lives into perspective but also to appreciate all the advantages we enjoy. The problems our recent ancestors had to face must have seemed insurmountable to them. If the dreadful diseases they had to endure can be overcome, then surely, with the correct approach, we can defeat our current health problems too.

In the nineteenth century when my great-great-grandmother was alive, the most common cause of death was an infectious disease such as tuberculosis, cholera, typhus or smallpox. Thanks to vaccinations, medications, sanitation, and education, we rarely see a life cut short by the sort of infection that killed her, at the age of 40, and her eldest son, who was 20, during the same week in 1868. It is highly likely that one of your ancestors also met an early death from an infection that could not be cured. We are very fortunate that these deadly diseases have almost been eliminated in the western world. To appreciate just how lucky we are, it is worth remembering the awful gory details of life, and death, before we had a National Health Service.

It is estimated that out of all the people who died in England between 1800 and 1850, one third of them died from tuberculosis.[1] The disease can infect the skin or the bones, but usually it is a bacterial infection of the lungs which causes pain, fever and massive damage to lung tissues. It also causes considerable weight loss, which led to its common name of 'consumption'. The disease spreads because each time an infected person coughs they expel bacteria into the air, and when someone else inhales that air they become infected. This disease killed 46,200 people in England in 1918 but thanks to antibiotics that number had tumbled to 256 in 2011.

Typhus is also a very infectious bacterial disease that is spread by body lice. The louse becomes diseased when it sucks the blood of an infected person. The bacteria grow inside the louse and eventually kill it, but not before the louse has moved on to someone else. The typhus-causing bacteria are in the faeces of the louse and when you scratch an itchy louse bite, you push the louse's infected faeces into your body. Someone with typhus suffers high fever, weakness and nausea leading to gangrene, delirium, coma and death by heart failure. When people had to live in crowded conditions and could not, or did not, wash frequently, the disease would spread rapidly. In the middle ages when the Spanish Army laid siege to Granada 3,000 men died in the fighting, but 17,000 died of typhus.[2] During Napoleon's retreat from Moscow, more French soldiers died from the disease than had died in the conflict. Thanks to vaccinations, insecticides and cleanliness, the developed world is now free from typhus.

On a similar theme, cholera is an infection of the intestines caused by drinking water contaminated by infected human excrement. Sometimes its effects were brutal. People could wake up in the morning feeling healthy, but suddenly become violently ill. Their skin would develop a horrible bluish tinge; they would produce huge quantities of milky-coloured, watery diarrhoea, thus making them severely dehydrated and causing death within hours.[3] Good sanitation has removed cholera from developed countries, but it still kills 100,000 people a year in the poorest parts of the world.

If you managed to avoid these ghastly diseases you may have fallen prey to smallpox, which was caused by an airborne virus, that would first attack the throat and skin. Fluid-filled, boil-like pustules would appear all over the skin, but as soon as the blood was infected the virus would spread rapidly throughout the body. If you survived you would probably be pockmarked, blind and have deformed limbs. It has been estimated that 200 years ago smallpox was killing 400,000 Europeans every year.[4] You will be relieved to know that you cannot catch Smallpox anymore because it has been completely eradicated. A worldwide programme of vaccinations made so many people immune that the virus could not find anybody to infect and it became extinct.

Good health for everyone?

We have come a long way since Victorian times and our victory over such awful diseases is one of mankind's greatest achievements. We should all be truly grateful that we live in modern times with clean water, sanitation, vaccines and medicines. The imagination, compassion and hard work of a very small number of wise people have made it possible for millions of other people to avoid the horrible, early death that befell so many of our recent ancestors.

The first antibiotic, penicillin, was discovered in 1928 by Alexander Fleming and it brought profound improvements in survival rates. After the Second World War the National Health Service was created which gave everybody free access to the best treatments that medicine could provide. The development of new drugs accelerated and doctors can now choose from a vast array of medicines to treat almost every illness. Within each group there are many drugs with slightly different actions. As an example, high blood pressure can be treated by drugs with a variety of effects:

- Removal of excess fluid by diuretics
- Dilation of the blood vessels
- Control of the hormones affecting blood pressure
- Reduction in the rate and force of heartbeats
- Direct action on the central control of blood pressure.

With so much progress, so many drug treatments and so many victories over fatal infections, it would be entirely logical to assume the entire population is in wonderful health and doctors and nurses have very little work to do. However, we all know that is not the case. The NHS is under severe pressure and the people of the United Kingdom are not healthy. Everybody is aware of the obesity crisis and that over-weight people are much more likely to develop diabetes, heart disease and cancer. We are told that 27% of the population are obese with a body mass index, BMI, of more than 30. A further 33% of people are overweight with a BMI between 25 and 30. We all know this is bad but what does it really mean?

If we assume there are 65 million people in the UK, 33% is 21.6 million people, who are on average 30 pounds overweight. There are 17.5 million obese people (27%), who are around 80 pounds overweight. When we multiply the number of people in each group by their excess weight and add the two groups together, we come to the mind-boggling result that the people of the United Kingdom are more than 2,000 million pounds overweight. I don't know how many Olympic swimming pools that much body fat would fill but it is a staggering burden for us all to be carrying around with us every day.

How is it possible that we have swapped the deadly diseases of the past for a whole range of new diseases of the present? The old diseases were infections passed from one person to another. The modern diseases cannot be caught from someone else but they are still at epidemic levels. The huge pressure under which the health service is struggling is caused by conditions like heart disease, diabetes, cancer, auto-immune diseases and a whole range of mental health problems. These conditions do not kill us quickly, like cholera, but they can still be truly awful. Type 2 diabetes, for instance, develops and progresses slowly but it can wreak havoc by destroying small blood vessels, which leads to kidney damage, blindness, amputation of the feet, dementia and an early death from heart disease.

Why are so many people ill? Why is the NHS struggling? Who is to blame? The culprit, in an extraordinary twist of irony, turns out to be the NHS itself. While the people working for it do a fantastic job, the NHS has become an enormous institution and it suffers from what I call 'institutionalised thinking'. It keeps doing what it has always done and the people at the top never stand back, take a good look at it and ask, "Are there any assumptions that we have made, and we adhere to, that might be completely wrong?"

The answer to that question is a resounding yes. The official dietary guidelines, which promote a low-fat and high-carbohydrate diet, are the problem. This dogma is enshrined in NHS policy, and prominent on their website, but it is the cause of the obesity crisis, the diabetes epidemic and the recent increase in dementia, to name but a few. These guidelines were first introduced in America in 1977 and Britain copied them in 1983. The following graph shows what has happened to obesity rates over time.

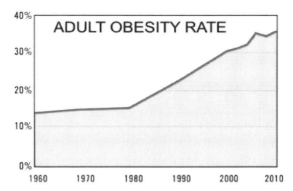

The relentless increase in weight gain, which immediately followed the introduction of the guidelines, could be a coincidence. A graph like this shows an association between two things but it doesn't prove that one thing caused the other. For proof of a cause, we need to identify a mechanism by which one thing causes the other and we need to be able to reverse the process by removing the cause. I will demonstrate both of those things in this book.

If you are overweight, you have probably been told to "eat less and move more". This is dreadful advice because it suggests that it is all your fault. It implies that you are overweight because you are greedy (eat too much) and lazy (don't move enough). It is categorically not your fault. The real reason people become overweight, and struggle to lose weight, is because they eat the wrong type of food. We have been told for over 30 years that we should base our meals on carbohydrate (bread, potatoes, pasta) and eat very little fat (butter, lard, cream, eggs, cheese and in meat). It has all gone catastrophically wrong because we have been lied to for years. However, while it is not your fault if you are too heavy, it is up to you to change things. You cannot expect someone else to fix this for you but I will help you to learn the truth. You will need to find motivation from within. During my career as an Olympic athlete, I learned how important the correct motivation is. You can achieve extraordinary things when you have goals that really matter to you. We can start with a little motivational game I like to play.

If I was to meet you and we got talking, I might ask you where you live. You would reply with the name of a town or village or maybe a street. I would then say, "No you don't." You would probably insist that you knew exactly where you lived and I would disagree with you. Before we reached the point where you walked away muttering that I was crazy, I would explain that what you are referring to is an address. You are thinking about the place where you keep your things and where you sleep at night. This is not strictly where you live because, from the moment you are born until the moment you die, you live your entire life inside your one and only body. Most of us stay in several different houses over the years but we all get just one body.

A lot of people are very house proud. They spend a great deal of time, money and effort turning their homes into warm, comfortable and attractive places, in which they are happy to stay. I wonder how many people put the same time, money and effort into maintaining the place where they really live? If it makes sense to maintain your boiler and plumbing to avoid having a sudden breakdown, then surely it makes sense to maintain your heart and all your arteries and veins? If you have a nice car with a finely tuned engine, would you put paraffin in the fuel tank? Petrol burns and paraffin burns, so why not use paraffin? You wouldn't do that because you know it would damage the engine. So why do so many people put highly-processed, refined and chemical-laden, food-like substances into their bodies and think it is alright?

Our bodies are entirely able to maintain good health if we look after them. We have an intricate network of controls and feedback mechanisms that operate automatically and constantly to maintain the optimum conditions for life. This is known as homeostasis. Examples of homeostasis include: the maintenance of our body temperature; regulation of our blood pressure; and the balance of our fluid levels. The condition of all our metabolic systems is continuously monitored by receptors and then adjusted by either nerve impulses or hormones. For example, it is important to maintain the correct level of sugar in the blood-stream and two hormones, with opposite effects, achieve this. One hormone, insulin, reduces blood sugar levels when they are too high and another hormone, glucagon, raises them when they are too low. If our bodies become too warm, nerve impulses activate the sweat glands and when we are too cold, different nerve impulses make our muscles shiver to produce warmth.

These and many other balancing mechanisms give us a lifetime of good health. We only become ill when something happens which pushes our normal, healthy condition so far out of line that our bodies cannot automatically restore the balance. Our immune system recognises, and then eliminates, bacteria and viruses that enter our bodies and we only become infected and ill when the invading bugs over-power our defensive response. Deficiencies in our diet, the ingestion of toxic chemicals or a lack of exercise will throw our system out of kilter and this disruption will lead to other types of disease.

Homeostasis is a remarkable system for maintaining good health. It evolved many millions of years ago and all living creatures benefit from their own version of it. From the sparrows in a garden, to the warthogs on the grasslands of Africa, every species can enjoy good health by living the way they are supposed to live. If lions eat meat, sheep eat grass, squirrels eat nuts and spiders eat flies, their homeostasis will keep them healthy. They all do very different things but they all prosper because they live in precisely the way they evolved to live.

Our species evolved to live in a certain way too but modern life has removed the necessity for us to behave as our ancestors did. There are four main things we need to do to allow homeostasis to keep us healthy and happy:

- Most importantly, we need to eat the right type of food.
- We need regular physical exercise.
- We need lots of sleep.
- We need to maintain low levels of stress.

As a species, we think we are quite clever. We can invent medicines to tackle almost any disease; we have doctors, nurses and hospitals to look after us but, sadly, we do not all live in perfect health. No matter how clever we think we are and no matter how much money we invest in health services, we still need to be true to ourselves.

The lion, sheep, squirrel and spider all know instinctively how to live their lives the way they should. There would be far less human illness if only we could do the same thing. So why can't we? To answer that, let's compare ourselves to garden birds. You don't have to be a 'twitcher' to notice common birds and recognise familiar varieties. Have you ever seen a sparrow, robin or blackbird that was too fat to fly and had to walk everywhere? No, neither have I. It doesn't happen because birds have a big advantage over us humans. Some of them gather in flocks and some are solitary but none of them have 'expert nutritional advice'. We have been terribly misled about what we should eat. I would go so far as to say we have been lied to repeatedly.

What are the three main influences on our lives? In no particular order, they are politics, religion and money. Would you be surprised to learn that the biggest influences on dietary advice over the last sixty years are not independent scientists but politics, religion and money? It is an extraordinary story in which our instincts and common sense have been usurped by the power of officialdom, the arrogance of ambitious scientists, the illogical beliefs of religious zealots and the advertising of profit-driven corporations. It is time to fight back; it is time for the truth.

Summary
- Free health care, via the NHS, costs £124 billion per year.
- The number of people who are ill continues to rise.
- Our recent ancestors died of infectious diseases but we are dying of metabolic diseases caused by our diet and lifestyle.
- The NHS promotes a diet which causes metabolic diseases.
- We can all be healthy if we eat and live the way we are supposed   to.

Chapter 2

MISINFORMATION, DOGMA AND GUIDELINES

If you are confused about what constitutes a healthy diet, you are not alone. Millions of people find it hard to distinguish reliable information from all the myths and misinformation. Newspapers are full of the latest studies suggesting coffee will make you live longer; or beetroot will prevent a heart attack; or three rashers of bacon will kill you. Where do all these ideas come from? How reliable is this information?

Mark Twain is reported to have said, "It is easier to fool people than to convince them that they have been fooled". I believe we have all been fooled by a combination of misinformation, mistakes and lies. As I said in Chapter 1, the hardest task for the human brain is to unlearn what we believe to be true. Many of us are confused about what we should eat to be healthy. We tend to get our information from newspapers and television, whose purpose is to write stories which will grab our attention rather than to explain the finer details of a scientific study. Most of the research in the field of nutrition is done by observational, or, as they are known in the world of science, epidemiological studies. By their very nature, these are the weakest type of scientific analysis because there are always so many variables to account for. If, for example, the people in one group admit to eating meat regularly and they are found to be less healthy than a group of vegetarians, how do we know it was meat that reduced their health? Someone who has decided to become vegetarian has decided that the quality of their food is important and they are likely to eat fresh, unprocessed food. Meat eaters in such a study will include people who eat lots of burgers at a fast food outlet. Is the meat in the burger the problem or is it the accompanying bun, fries and large fizzy drink that are to blame? The only way to be sure is to compare groups of people who only eat fresh, unprocessed vegetables with people who only eat fresh, unprocessed meat.

A major problem with all observational studies on nutrition is the accuracy of the data. The researchers rely on food frequency questionnaires, where the participants have to remember what they have had to eat. Can you remember precisely what you ate a week last Thursday? No, neither can I.

The only genuine success, achieved by observational studies, is the link between smoking and lung cancer. Researchers discovered that regular smokers were 16 times more likely to develop lung cancer than non-smokers. When one activity makes something else 16 times more likely to happen, it is hugely significant. This observation led to the detailed studies which confirmed that cigarette smoke is the most common cause of lung cancer.

However, most of the recent observational studies used by the World Health Organisation (WHO) to warn us that certain foods should be limited, or avoided, have found a relationship to disease of about 1.5 to 1. I do not understand how such a tiny increase in risk can be statistically relevant. Observational studies just cannot be that accurate. In order to classify the significance of observational research, a system called Grade was developed.[1] The Grade system for ranking the relevance of studies based on epidemiology requires a minimum of a fivefold increased risk before the observation can be regarded as the cause of the problem. The 16 fold risk of smoking is way beyond the realms of random variables but a 1.5 risk could easily occur by chance. The World Health Organisation has signed up to this system but frequently ignores it. If the World Health Organisation cannot get this right, what hope is there for journalists and the public to grasp the relevance of these details?

With all the contradictory information that is available in the media and online, it seems reasonable to revert to logic to find our way through this maze. The ability to apply logical thinking to a situation usually leads to a correct idea or decision. However, it is important to realise that we need good information to be able to make a logical decision as I will explain in the following example.

For thousands of years, everybody believed that the sun moved around the earth. It is logical to think so because every day the sun rises in the east, it arcs across the sky and sets in the west. It is then dark for about the same time that it was light, before the sun comes up again in the east. It would seem obvious to assume the Sun goes around the Earth – except that we know it does not. Something is happening that we cannot feel nor easily see. The Earth is spinning on its axis and this makes it look as if the Sun is moving.

It was a Polish astronomer called Nicolaus Copernicus who first observed this phenomenon in 1543. A few decades later the Italian astronomer, Galileo, published a book supporting the idea that the Sun is at the centre of our solar system and the Earth spins on its axis. We all know that he was right but the authorities at the time did not like his theory because it threatened their religious beliefs and positions of power. Instead of congratulating Galileo on his work, they put him under house arrest for the rest of his life. Their religion was more important to them than science and they insisted that the Earth was the centre of the solar system.

Many of the myths and lies we are told about health and food have an element of 'the Sun goes around the Earth', by which I mean, something may appear to be logical but it turns out to be completely wrong. In reality, there is something else going on that you cannot easily see and there are many examples of this throughout the book. Sadly, there are also recent examples of open-minded scientists who have challenged the dogma of the authorities and have been censored for it. I will explain more about this in Chapter 9.

Let's look at an observational study to see how misleading they can be. In the following diagram, there are 12 separate readings. The data is completely reliable; it has been verified on many occasions.

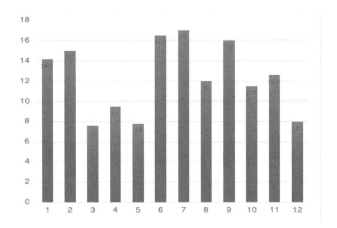

For now, I am deliberately hiding what has been measured here. The results appear to be completely random but there is a factor among them which makes them more interesting. Eight of the 12 readings contain something to which I will give the letter R. The four which do not contain R are the readings numbered 2, 6, 7 and 9 along the bottom of the diagram. We can see that these four have the largest response, or effect, because they extend higher than the other measurements.

If we separate the four readings without R from the eight with R and produce an average for the two groups, we can clearly see, in the diagram below, that whatever R is, it makes a considerable difference. In fact, the difference is 35%.

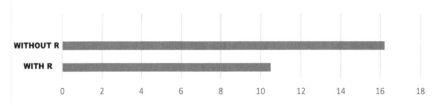

If this was a study of a horrible disease and R was my special potion to reduce the occurrence of this illness by 35%, I suspect I would sell a lot of bottles of potion. Many people would trust that R was producing a significant benefit as demonstrated by these diagrams but there is actually no proof of any benefit here.

The 12 pieces of data in the first diagram are actually the months of the year and the readings are the average hours of light during each day of the month. To make it look random, I arranged the months alphabetically instead of chronologically. The mysterious factor R is, in fact, the letter 'r'. It is simply a coincidence that the only months without the letter 'r' in their names are the four consecutive months of the summer: May, June, July and August. (Or winter, if you are in the Southern hemisphere, where you would have the least daylight.) We know for certain that the way we spell the name of a month has nothing to do with how many hours of sunshine there are in that month. A convincing graph, appearing to show that one thing causes another thing, is never proof of causation because it might be nothing more than a simple coincidence. In this example, I deliberately chose the letter R because I knew it would produce a result that looks convincing. If I had chosen the letter A instead, there would be no difference between the two groups because January, February, March, April, May and August contain A and the other six months do not.

The purpose of this example is twofold. If the data above had been for something we do not understand, it would be easy to think that the chart proved that R had a profound effect. A correlation cannot prove anything by itself because it can always be coincidence. However, good scientists would look at such a chart and investigate further. There are three things that can be done:

- Try to find a mechanism by which R exerts its apparent effect and thus be able to explain how it happens.
- Run a randomised, controlled trial that either eliminates, or adds, one specific factor to an otherwise comparable group and see if it exerts its effect across one group but not the other.
- Devise experiments that attempt to disprove what the chart suggests.

That is what good scientists would do but sadly, in the world of nutrition and the dietary guidelines, this is not always the case. (This is how you have a trial which is both randomised and controlled, in case you are wondering. The organisers of a trial would recruit, say, 1,000 people to take part. They use a method to allocate these people randomly into two groups of 500, so that there is no deliberate selection of participants. What the two groups then do, or eat, is carefully controlled. These studies are referred to as RCTs in scientific reports and they are usually the most reliable method of conducting a trial.)

The second point about my example is to emphasise the effect of bias. We all exhibit some sort of bias in our opinions because of our beliefs and experiences. In the field of research, there is something called confirmation bias, where we pay more attention to something that confirms what we already think. I had realised that R would produce a striking result while A would not. I used bias to try to convince you of something that could not be shown by selecting letters randomly. Complicated observational studies are prone to the bias of the researchers, whether it occurs deliberately or subconsciously. Let's bear this in mind while we look at the events that led to the publication of the American dietary guidelines in 1977, which Britain copied a few years later.

The dietary guidelines
Our national dietary guidelines are based on the incorrect idea that saturated fat causes heart disease [2]. We are told, therefore, to reduce the amount of fat we eat and, to do this and avoid hunger, we must increase the amount of carbohydrate. We have been advised to eat a high-carbohydrate, low-fat diet since 1983 and the whole purpose of this advice was to reduce the risk of heart disease. The medical profession had never come across heart disease until 100 years ago. The first heart attack (myocardial infarction) to be recorded as such was in the USA in 1921. (Heart disease would have existed long before this but doctors were generally unaware of it.) By 1930 there had been 3,000 more deaths caused by heart attacks. Doctors were very worried about this new disease but did not know what caused it, nor how to prevent it.

Autopsies showed that the victims of a heart attack had swellings in some of their arteries and these swellings, known as plaques, were found to contain large concentrations of cholesterol.

They assumed, therefore, cholesterol was the cause of heart disease. (This, of course, is typical 'the Sun goes around the Earth' thinking, but we will look at that in more detail in the Chapter 5.) An American researcher called Ancel Keys is at the root of all our dietary problems. He was convinced that high levels of cholesterol were to blame for the increasing epidemic of heart disease in middle-aged and older men. He was aware that people who ate a high level of fat in their diet tended to have slightly higher levels of cholesterol transported in the blood. From a variety of countries, he collated information about the number of people suffering heart disease and the amount of fat eaten in a diet typical of those countries. In 1953 he presented the following graph of his findings:

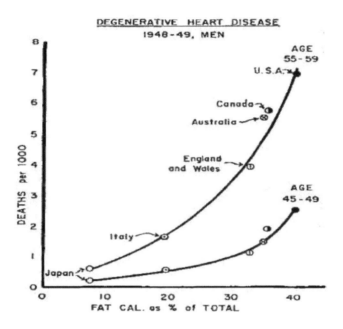

This is known as the Keys' Six Countries Study and it looks very convincing. It clearly shows that death from degenerative heart disease increases as dietary fat increases. A lot of people began to agree with Keys after seeing this graph. However, most of them were unaware of that thing called confirmation bias. The information Keys had used was available for 22 countries but he chose to plot the results of only six: the six countries which perfectly fitted the result he wanted to achieve.

Other researchers, Yerushalmy and Hilleboe, produced a paper in 1957 with the information from all 22 countries. It is clear from the diagram below that any correlation between fat and heart disease is far less convincing than Keys would have had us believe. If we compare Norway (17), for example, with the United States (22), we can see they consume very similar amounts of fat but the US has more than twice as much heart disease. Also, if we pick six countries to suit our purpose we can show the opposite effect. A line drawn between 17, 15, 9, 20, 2 and 11 would suggest heart disease increases when there is less fat in the diet.

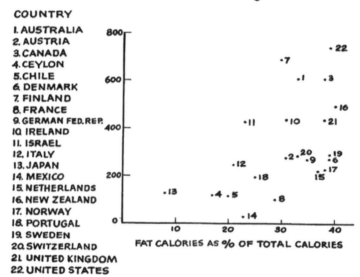

FIG. 13   Mortality from Arteriosclerotic and Degenerative Heart Disease and percent of total calories from fat--Males age 55-59, 1950

Fig. 13.   Yerushalmy, J. and Hilleboe, H. E.[35]

When the President of the United States, Dwight Eisenhower, had a heart attack in 1955 everybody started to panic. Politicians and doctors became determined to find the cause and cure for this silent killer. Ancel Keys, who was already well-known, wasted no time in telling everybody to eat a low-fat and low-cholesterol diet. Eisenhower's doctor, Paul Dudley White, advised him to eat less fat and cholesterol but he did not ask him to stop smoking cigarettes. (The connection between smoking and heart disease had not been made at this time.) On his new diet, the President's weight increased and he suffered six more heart attacks before he finally died of one. (The low-fat, low-cholesterol diet that is still official advice made him heavier and did nothing to stop further cardiac problems.)

Keys was very keen to prove his theory once and for all, so he launched an ambitious study of seven countries, which he and his fellow researchers visited. After two years of preparation, the observations began in 1958 and the results were published 12 years later in 1970. From all this work he concluded it was not total dietary fat but saturated fat intake that was the cause of heart disease. Ancel Keys was a very intelligent man: he had a Degree in Economics, a Master's degree in Zoology, a PhD in Oceanography and another PhD in Physiology. Despite all of this, he allowed his bias to dominate his work in the field of nutrition, for which he had no qualifications.

In her fascinating book, *The Big Fat Surprise*, investigative journalist Nina Teicholz explains, in detail, all the problems and flaws in the collection of data for the Seven Countries Study. True to form, Keys carefully chose countries he believed would give the results he was hoping for, but he also made some fundamental mistakes. For example, he studied a devoutly Christian community during Lent, when, of course, nobody eats the same food they consume for the rest of the year. There were also issues with his assessment of how much saturated fat different foods contain, which is a big problem when he blamed saturated fat for thousands of heart attack deaths. Also, he classified cake and ice cream as fat. They both contain fat but by far the biggest ingredient is carbohydrate, largely in the form of sugar. He was finding that people who ate lots of cake and ice cream were more likely to have heart disease; however, he decided to lay the blame on fat, whilst ignoring the effect of sugar. He also thought that plant fats were superior to animal fats because he believed they contained less saturated fat. He praised communities with diets high in olive oil over those consuming considerable amounts of pork. He didn't appear to know that a tablespoon of olive oil has more than three times the fat and a third more saturated fat than a pork chop.

Other eminent scientists at the time were publishing their own research into the cause of heart disease. Yerushalmy and Hilleboe, whose graph of 22 countries we have already seen, examined the effects on health of all the major food groups, rather than just concentrating on fat. They discovered that the relationship between the consumption of fat and all causes of death was negative. In other words, the more dietary fat people ate, the less likely they were to die of any cause. They also discovered a negative correlation between the amount of animal protein eaten and death from other causes. According to these two researchers, it is wrong to believe that the reduction of animal meat and fat in our diets will improve our health.

Professor John Yudkin was a British researcher whose work had shown that sugar was a far more likely cause of heart disease than dietary fat. In 1972 he published a book called *Pure, White and Deadly* in which he explained why the consumption of sugar was leading to a greatly increased incidence of heart disease. He also explained why sugar was certainly involved in tooth decay, probably involved in obesity, diabetes and liver disease and possibly involved in gout and some cancers. (As we will see later, all these things are true.)

Ancel Keys' unflinching belief that saturated fat causes heart disease, led him to produce biased research. However, I believe that his arrogance was even worse than his bias. He vehemently attacked Yudkin and Hilleboe and disparaged their work as if they were fools. Keys attacked Yudkin so aggressively that it ruined his career. After so much criticism, Yudkin was unable to get funding for more research, despite being a brilliant scientist ahead of his time. It is tragic to think that if Yudkin had been the arrogant bully, instead of Keys, we would probably not have an obesity epidemic across the world today.

While all this was going on, it became apparent that many Americans were suffering from malnutrition and housewives were complaining that food was too expensive. A select committee of senators was created under the leadership of George McGovern and from 1968 to 1977 they listened to evidence from a variety of nutritional experts. There were plenty of people who disagreed with Keys and his hypothesis on fat, but he criticised them all and bullied his way into the minds of the committee members. He persuaded them that saturated fat, which is found much more in animal foods than plant-based foods, was causing the ever-rising rate of heart disease and its consumption should be greatly reduced. It was inevitable that, if people were going to eat less fat, they would have to eat more carbohydrate to obtain their energy. The high-carbohydrate, low-fat diet became enshrined in the official guidelines and the entire population was encouraged to follow this doctrine. Nobody on the committee gave any serious thought to the potentially negative outcomes of such a huge change in eating habits. They simply decided that if fat was bad, they would have to recommend the only alternative. The committee was full of law-making Senators but they failed to appreciate the Law of Unintended Consequences.

The new rationale was seen by the politicians involved as an opportunity. If everybody was going to eat bread and cereals instead of meat, food bills would become cheaper and to make sure this happened they gave subsidies to farmers growing wheat and similar crops. This gave the farmers the impetus to rip out hedgerows and create enormous fields of single crops that could be harvested on an industrial scale (with terrible consequences to wildlife). Naturally, the livestock farmers were not happy and the senators representing them demanded a compromise. It was agreed, therefore, to include the term 'lean meat' in the dietary guidelines that became official policy in America in 1977. We are still advised to eat only 'lean meat' and most people would assume it has been proven to be healthier. However, nobody has ever produced a scrap of scientific evidence to show any benefit for lean meat over more fatty cuts of meat. It was never science; it was always just a political compromise made by a committee that was dominated by a biased and arrogant scientist.

The official dietary guidelines, which were copied by Britain in 1983 and most of the world shortly after, recommended that people should reduce overall fat consumption to 30% of total energy and reduce saturated fat consumption to 10% of total energy. The shortfall would be replaced by increasing carbohydrate intake to 60% of energy. Properly conducted, randomised control trials (as opposed to observational studies used by Keys) were available at the time but none of them were referred to by the McGovern Select Committee, nor by the British authorities when they followed suit. One of these studies, by Woodhill and Palmer, tested the recommendation for 10% saturated fat and discovered a higher rate of death among the group on the lowest intake of fat.[3] Combining the results from all the other trials confirmed there was no benefit to the low-fat diet. All of this was ignored because the committee was motivated by politics and not by good science.

One of the people who testified before the committee, and whose testimony was ignored, was a British doctor, surgeon and Royal Navy Captain called Thomas Cleave. He believed that good nutrition was essential to good health and his research had convinced him that too much carbohydrate was the cause of many diseases. He published a book about this called *The Saccharine Disease*. During his testimony, when asked about meat and animal foods, he said, "For a modern disease to be related to an old-fashioned food is one of the most ludicrous things I have ever heard in my life". When Doctor Cleave referred to meat as an 'old-fashioned food', he did not mean that it was no longer fashionable: he meant that humans have been eating it for a very long time. It was entirely logical to him that a food our ancestors have consumed for millions of years cannot suddenly become the cause of a modern disease. Sadly, the committee did not appreciate the importance of 'old-fashioned food'.

Summary:

- Research on nutrition usually involves information from unreliable, food-frequency questionnaires in an observational study. These studies cannot prove that one thing causes another thing to happen and they are often affected by researcher bias.
- The official dietary guidelines were based on biased, observational studies carried out by one man, Ancel Keys, with an unshakeable belief that saturated fat caused heart disease. There was no real evidence that this was true and there is still no evidence.
- Politicians took advantage of Keys' theory to increase grain production, which lowered food prices and boosted exports. But, because they did not listen to concerned scientists, they set in motion the worldwide obesity epidemic.
- Good scientists, who disagreed with the saturated fat hypothesis, were silenced.

Chapter 3

EVOLUTION AND WHY IT MATTERS

Of all the creatures on the planet, it can be said that humans have the best brains. This may be true because our brains are large compared to our body size, or it may be true because of the exceptional connectivity and processing power that our 100 billion neurones provide. It is definitely true if we want to live the life of a human. If, for some reason, you wanted to live the life of, say, a Great White Shark, our brains are hopeless. The Great White can smell a drop of blood in sea water from over 100 metres away because of its exceptionally well-developed olfactory bulb. If the Great White Shark had a sense of humour, it would laugh at our pathetic sense of smell. Sharks, of course, don't have a sense of humour because their brains are nowhere near complex enough. However, they are very well adapted to the life they live because their evolution concentrated on just one way to find food.

The need to eat was also responsible for the evolution of our brains and we developed more complex brains because of the way our ancestors found their food. One of the problems with any theory of evolution is that the people involved didn't keep any diaries for us to read; however, all the facts suggest that a period of climate change set off a sequence of events, which eventually gave us the most complex brains on the planet. It is truly ironic that climate change gave us the brains to develop the complex civilisations, tools and machines that scientists believe will cause a further change in the climate, which may destroy us!

We all inherit the genes that make us what we are from our mother and father, who in turn inherited their genes from their parents, and so on, back through the generations and back through the centuries. If we assume that 25 is the average age when a man and woman have a child, we get four generations in every century and, therefore, forty generations in a thousand years. Everybody has a father and mother, so you have a direct line of about 100 male and female ancestors going back to the time of the Roman Empire. So how far back does this line go?

Genetic research has shown that our nearest cousins in the animal world are the chimpanzees, and both we and they evolved from a common, tree-living ancestor about seven million years ago. Experts believe a major change in the climate caused a huge loss of trees in the African rainforest, which led to the formation of open grasslands, and because of this our ancestors were forced to adapt and change. They stopped living in the trees like other apes and began to walk on two feet instead of four. Their diet had to change too and the groups that survived ate a variety of new foods. During those seven million years the brain of the chimpanzee has remained roughly the same but our brain has trebled in size.

The process that made us what we are today emerged about two million years ago. That is when people evolved who were clearly like the humans of today and, with that time scale, you and I are descendants of about 100,000 generations of two-footed, human-like mammals. An enormous amount of adaptation to the environment must have happened through so many ancestors and this information has been passed down to you and me in our genes.

What differences have occurred between us and the chimpanzees during all that time? What are the main changes that we have undergone in the last few million years? We have straightened our spines and hips so we stand and walk upright; we have lost our body hair and developed sweat glands so that we are very good at losing excess heat; and we have developed much bigger and better brains.

What did we do to make these changes happen? Instead of sitting in a tree reaching out for the fruit and nuts around us, we were forced to search for food when the trees disappeared. Standing up straight and walking on two feet was faster and more efficient than using all four limbs, the way chimpanzees do. As we became more upright, we became taller and could see further, which helped us to spot both food and danger.

We do not possess the enzymes to digest grass and there are not many other plants growing on a large expanse of grassland we could eat. However, the animals that do eat grass provide a very nutritious meal as long as you can catch them. Hunting animals on the African Savanna a million years ago is what made us what we are today. The changes we had to make to survive are clear in the DNA we have inherited. We probably started eating animal flesh as scavengers: making the most of leftovers from a big cat's kill. It is a logical idea and explains why the acid in our stomach is a stronger acid than other primates. The only other animals with equally acidic stomachs are all scavengers.

The ancestors of lions, tigers and cheetahs were busy catching the ancestors of gazelle and impala, but meat is meat and they were quite happy to eat our ancestors too. Big cats don't like to get too hot and they hunt in the early morning or evening when it is cooler. Early humans realised they were much less likely to be eaten themselves if they went hunting for food in the middle of the day. A typical grass-eating animal, like the antelopes of today, would be chewing grass for hours whilst watching out for lions and tigers. They evolved to sprint away from a big cat but had no need to keep running for a long time. They either got away or they didn't. Both they and the big cats were very poor at losing body heat and would sprint for a few seconds and then pant, like a domestic dog, to cool down.

We couldn't sprint fast enough to catch any of these animals, so we took a different approach. We would work in a group and chase one animal in the heat of the day.[1] Our prey would easily get away at first but we would catch up to it again before it had time to cool down. It would run away again and again but each time it would be getting hotter. Eventually, it would collapse from heat exhaustion and we could walk up to it and enjoy a very large and nutritious meal. Our bodies adapted to this way of life because all of our ancestors were using the same method to hunt. The Bushmen of the Kalahari still hunt for food in exactly this way. The animals we hunted didn't need to change because the herds they lived in survived well by sprinting away from danger.

These early humans had not yet developed any tools but they only needed a rock or pointed stick to finish off an animal that had collapsed from heat stroke. We avoided heat stroke by losing our body hair and developing extensive sweat glands. Sweating by itself does not cause cooling of the body: it is evaporation of water from the surface of the skin that does so. Body hair keeps warmth in but also restricts evaporation from the skin. So, the combination of hair loss and sweating allowed us to develop the ability to run in the midday heat. This is an ability we still have today, as demonstrated by elite marathon runners. In fact, humans are one of the very few animals on the planet with the ability to travel long distances on foot. Horses and wolves, which belong to a group of animals called ungulates, are the only other creatures with a similar ability. However, they cannot lose body heat as we do. Our loss of hair and the development of sweat glands are a clear indication that our ancestors had to run and walk long distances to catch the food they needed to survive.[2] We could not have developed these exceptional abilities if our diet consisted of plants.

When our ancestors caught an animal they would eat all of it. There is no chance they ate just the lean meat and left everything else. They would eat the liver, heart, brains and fat, as well as the muscles. Indeed, fat was the most precious part. There are many references to fat in ancient literature: 'living off the fat of the land'; 'kill the fatted calf'. Animal fat provides the most important nutrients for the human brain because 60% of the structure of the brain consists of fat molecules (excluding water).[3] The most important fats for the brain are omega-3 fatty acids; eicosapentaenoic acid (EPA); and docosahexaenoic acid (DHA). These are only found in animal food sources. DHA makes up about 14% of our brain structure, and therefore, our ancestors must have had a prolonged and rich source of this essential nutrient.

While fatty acids in the brain strongly suggest our ancestors were primarily carnivores, the evidence from vitamin B12 makes it irrefutable. Among other things, vitamin B12 is responsible for the production of red blood cells, as well as the myelin sheath which covers all of our nerve fibres. Animals with both a circulatory and nervous system must absorb adequate levels of B12 in order to live. Plants have neither of these systems and, therefore, contain none of this essential nutrient. If herbivores need it but do not eat it, how do they survive? Vitamin B12 is made by the bacteria that thrive in the rumen, or caecum, of plant-eating animals. The human digestive tract does not contain an equivalent compartment. We possess B12-producing bacteria in our colons, but by a quirk of evolutionary fate, we cannot absorb any of it from the large intestine. All of the vitamin B12 we make goes down the toilet. We can only absorb this nutrient from the small intestine and the bacteria living there cannot make it. Evolution could not have allowed this situation to develop unless our ancestors were eating a regular supply of B12-rich animal foods.

As we evolved, our brains became bigger and they needed considerably more energy. According to a metabolic constant known as Kleiber's Law, when one organ in an animal's body starts to use more energy it is necessary for another organ to use less. It was our digestive tract that grew smaller while our brains enlarged. In order to absorb the fats we needed for a growing brain, from shrinking intestines, we must have been eating nutrient-dense, easily-absorbed foods. Animals are the only possible source of such nourishment. Other primates that eat a plant-based diet, like gorillas, have large intestines and small brains.

One of the reasons we have such well-developed brains has only been discovered recently and it is all to do with running after that nutritious food. Successfully hunting an animal, until it collapsed from heat exhaustion, required several different skills. Our ancestors had to work as a group, which required communication and cooperation. They also needed spatial awareness, a sense of direction and memory. These are all functions of a well-developed brain. It turns out that all the running, walking and chasing developed the brain directly.

It has now been proven that the contraction of muscles during physical exercise produces a hormone called Irisin. When this hormone reaches the brain, it triggers the production of chemical compounds called neurotrophic factors.[4] (Neuro means nerve and trophic means growth, so a neurotrophic factor is a chemical which causes nerve cells to grow.) When you create a memory inside your brain, a physical connection is built between two brain cells. You need to have nerve-growth factors present for this connection to be made because they are the chemicals which make it happen. The human brain is superior to that of other animals, partly because it is larger, but mainly because it has far more connections between cells than the brains of other creatures. All the physical exercise, the running, walking, hunting and gathering, which our ancestors did every day for hundreds of thousands of years, produced high levels of nerve growth factors. These molecules allowed all that superior connectivity to be formed and for our brains to become more complex. Nerve growth factors do not make the brain more intelligent all by themselves but they do put the brain into the optimum condition for creating and retrieving memories and for critical thinking.

Our distant ancestors had to solve a wide range of problems when finding and catching food. All the running they did, in pursuit of their next meal, primed their brains to remember their experiences and to think how best to use those experiences. Chasing after their dinner, which involved solving problems and producing nerve growth factors, was the process that put humans on the evolutionary road to the intelligence and brain power we enjoy today.

Carl Cotman, of San Diego University, was one of the first scientists to show, in 2002, that physical exercise is responsible for the production of the neurotrophic factors which greatly improve the formation of memories. During the last decade many scientists from around the world have confirmed this to be true and we will see details of this in later chapters. Despite this indisputable body of evidence, some people find it hard to believe that chemicals produced by muscular contraction can have such a profound effect upon the brain. To some minds, it seems much more logical that thought and concentration would be the driving force behind improved brain function. That misconception can easily be dealt with by looking much further back in time.

When life first began on Earth, about four hundred million years ago, organisms were very small and simple. At first, as they drifted through water absorbing nutrients around them, some attached themselves to surfaces and absorbed food that drifted by. Eventually, they grew more complex and when the first nerve cells evolved, these creatures could move themselves in search of food. Nerve cells provide the impulse for the contractions which produce movement. Being able to go in search of food meant much better nutrition, which provided the energy to develop a better system of nerves, which in turn provided better movement. So, from the very beginning of life, movement and the nervous system have always been complimentary parts of the same process. They have always been totally interlinked and when you understand this, it becomes logical that just as the nervous system produces movement, it is movement that enhances the nervous system.

To understand this point further you could consider a tree. Trees are magnificent living organisms: they can live for hundreds of years; they respond to the seasons; they absorb carbon dioxide from the air; keep the carbon for growth; and give back the oxygen we all need for life. They can produce beautiful blossom and provide fruit or nuts. They can do all these things, but they have absolutely no nervous system for the very simple reason that they don't go anywhere. No movement means no nervous system.

On the Great Barrier Reef there is a creature called a Sea Squirt, which is born with a spinal cord and a primitive brain. It swims along the coral searching for a place to live and, when it finds a suitable location, it puts down roots. Once it is safely attached, the Sea Squirt consumes its own brain. For most of its life it looks much more like a plant than an animal and, because it is not moving, it has no use for a brain. The nervous system provides movement and in return movement provides the nervous system.

Nowadays we tend to regard our brains as a processor of thoughts and a control centre which is separate from the rest of our bodies. This is not true. Our brains are simply a highly-evolved extension of the nervous system which still controls our movements and still requires movement to function properly. Our brains evolved because of our circumstances but, of course, so did the rest of us. Our species has spent 98% of its existence living as hunter-gatherers and our genetic code is hunter-gatherer code. Almost everybody on the planet now lives a more modern lifestyle based upon a constant and reliable supply of food from agriculture and a system of monetary reward for what is often specialised work, in a narrow field of endeavour. Human life has changed much more quickly than our genetic make-up ever could and this divergence between what we are, and how we live, is at the root of many of the physical and emotional problems that are now so common.

In the most remote parts of the world there are still a few small groups of people who have never changed. They continue to live the hunter-gatherer life that made us all what we are today. They include the Kung, Ache, Baka, Aka, Bofi, San, Hadza and Efe tribes. Some of these people live in jungles, while others reside in deserts but because they are sufficiently remote from modern developments, they have been able to continue to live in much the same way as our ancestors used to do. The survival of these tribes has given scientists a fantastic opportunity to study our development and evolution. Some people may assume that these almost naked, nomadic groups are simply primitive savages, but they are invariably friendly and generous people, who have allowed anthropologists to live with them with for long periods of time to study their way of life. Hunter-gatherer tribes believe that everybody in the group is of equal importance and scientists therefore refer to them as 'egalitarian societies'.[5] There may be hundreds of people in a tribe but they usually live in groups of about 20 to 30 because this is the sort of number that can function well together. They have no appointed leaders and all their major decisions are made by talking things through until there is agreement. People from the developed world have suggested that this approach is very time-consuming and inefficient, but the hunter-gatherers' response is to ask what could possibly be a more important use of your time?

This egalitarianism is particularly interesting because our nearest cousins, the chimpanzees, live in groups with a clear social hierarchy which is dominated by an alpha male. Anthropologists now believe that our resistance to being dominated was a key factor driving the evolutionary emergence of human consciousness, language, kinship and social organisation. The most enjoyable and rewarding aspects of modern life usually involve social gatherings where we interact with each other respectfully and in a mutually beneficial way. Hundreds of thousands of years ago our ancestors realised that they were all far better off if they cooperated with each other and that everybody had a contribution to make to the group. Research has shown that people nowadays are happiest when they are part of a loving, caring family; they have a social group of about 20 real friends; they feel valued for what they do; they are not too hung-up by what they possess; and are willing to help other people. In other words, happy people live a life which has been normal for our species for the last million years.

Hunter-gatherers have little interest in possessions and are happy to share what they have with the rest of their group. They do not usually store food and therefore must find new food every day. However, as soon as they have enough, they go back to their camp and sit around the fire talking to each other. They typically work for two or three hours fewer each day than someone in an industrial society and, of course, they sleep throughout the night. Their babies are breast-fed for a couple of years; they receive a great deal of physical contact and their cries are always attended to quickly. Children can play freely with boys and girls of different ages all day long and this continues until they are adults. (We will see how important this is in Chapter 15.) The adults in the group can all be relied upon to look after and help any of the children.

Other interesting findings from the study of hunter-gatherer groups involve their health. While infections and accidents cause a higher percentage of deaths than we see in the developed world, these people are remarkably free from the diseases of modern society. Mental illnesses like clinical depression and schizophrenia are almost non-existent and there is absolutely no evidence of child abuse. Obesity, heart disease and diabetes are metabolic abnormalities that just do not happen to people who live a life that is normal for our species: a life of daily exercise and sufficient sleep, with a diet of unprocessed food, in a community of people who all care for each other and who have enough leisure time to enjoy each other's company.

I am not suggesting for a moment that any of us should form communes and wander the countryside living on what we can find, as if the hunter-gatherer lifestyle would be a blissful utopia. However, I am saying that we are incredibly foolish if we ignore the evidence that these remaining hunter-gatherer people provide. They live happy, healthy lives which are completely free from modern life-style diseases because they live the way we all evolved to live. Millions of people in the developed world have become abnormal and suffer physical and mental ill-health because our modern lives are too far removed from our evolution. There is no great secret to health and happiness; we need to incorporate normal human behaviour into our lives and become a normal member of our own species.

Summary:
- We evolved into what we are today by a lengthy process of chasing after animals and eating them.
- The chasing produced large numbers of brain-enhancing molecules.
- Essential fats, from which our brains are created, came from the animals we ate.
- Our exceptional ability to run long distances, especially in hot weather, is proof of our specific evolution.
- We were successful as a species because of our diet and also because we lived in egalitarian groups, committed to helping each other.

Chapter 4

HOW TO LOSE WEIGHT WITHOUT FEELING HUNGRY

When people want to lose weight they usually go on a 'diet', which involves eating less food than normal. It is easy to understand the logic: if we consume fewer calories than we use each day, the shortfall will have to come from our fat stores and this will lead to weight loss. Thousands of people have lost weight by this method. Unfortunately, nearly all of them have put the weight back on because this type of semi-starvation is not sustainable. It seems obvious that eating less will reduce our weight and keep it off but that is not the case. This apparently logical idea is wrong because something more complex is happening. Our weight is not controlled by counting calories: it is controlled by hormones and metabolism.

Everything that happens inside our bodies is carefully regulated by the wonderful system of homeostasis. If we eat less food than we need for a day, we simply take what we need from storage. If we eat less food than we need for a month, as we would on a restrictive diet, our bodies think there is a famine and homeostasis reduces our metabolic rate to save energy. Rather like turning down the thermostat on the central heating to save gas, our internal systems reduce our normal temperature slightly to save energy and as a result we feel cold. We also feel lethargic and distinctly hungry. The continuous sense of hunger requires a great deal of willpower to resist day after day. Eventually we all give in to temptation and eat more because feeling cold, lethargic and hungry all the time makes us miserable.

At some point, whether we reach our target weight or not, we decide that we have done well and we can go back to eating normally. The problem is that 'eating normally' is what made us overweight in the first place, but now we have slowed down our metabolism. Our bodies are using less energy for daily requirements than before and when we start eating the way we used to, we store all that extra energy as fat. The weight, which we have slowly and painstakingly lost, piles back on. Many people end up on a rollercoaster of going on a diet, losing weight, putting it back on and going on another diet. There are some cynical people who think this is the business model of the well-known weight loss organisations: they will never run out of customers if weight loss is only temporary.

Semi starvation

This problem of weight loss and gain ought to be well known because during the Second World War researchers at the University of Minnesota began an experiment on the psychology and physiology of human starvation and hunger [1]. The subjects were 36 conscientious objectors of various weights. These men were semi-starved for 24 weeks. They ate nearly 1,600 calories a day of foods chosen to represent those available in European famine areas: whole-wheat bread; potatoes; cereals; considerable amounts of turnips and cabbage; token amounts of meat and dairy. (This experiment would not be allowed nowadays because it would be regarded as unethical.)

The men lost an average of one pound of body fat per week over the first 12 weeks, but that slowed to quarter of a pound per week over the following 12. This was not their only physiological reaction: their extremities swelled, their hair fell out and wounds healed slowly. They felt cold continuously as their metabolism slowed. Even worse than these were the psychological effects. The men became depressed, lethargic and irritable. They threw tantrums. They lost their libido. They thought obsessively about food, day and night. The Minnesota researchers called this 'semi-starvation neurosis'. Two of them had breakdowns: one with talk of suicide and threats of violence and he was committed to the psychiatric ward. The personality deterioration of the other man ended in two attempts at self-mutilation.

When the period of imposed starvation ended, the subjects were allowed to eat more calories, but were restricted as to how many. A group of them, under continued observation, was then allowed to eat until they were full, which was surprisingly hard to achieve. The men ate huge amounts of food: up to 10,000 calories a day. They regained weight and fat with remarkable speed. After 20 weeks of recovery they averaged 50% more body fat than they had had when the experiment began. The researchers called this post-starvation obesity.

Seventy years ago this study showed that failing to eat enough food each day, for an extended period of time, resulted in weight loss. However, it also caused a range of dire physical and psychological problems making it unsustainable as a diet. The rapid and considerable weight gain afterwards makes a restricted diet not just difficult but also futile.

The calorie counting myth

Is it possible to lose weight and keep it off without willpower, hunger and lethargy? Yes it is, but before we get to that we need some basic information. We are always told to count the calories in our food and that weight loss comes from consuming fewer calories than we use. This is referred to as the 'Calories in – Calories out' method of weight loss, or the CICO diet. In early 2018 the Government-backed organisation, Public Health England (PHE), issued guidance on what we should eat, in its attempts to reverse the obesity epidemic. They proclaimed that all adults should eat 400 calories for breakfast, 600 calories for lunch and 600 calories for dinner, with 100 to 200 calories in snacks twice a day.

In my opinion, the nutrition department of Public Health England is one of the most misguided organisations that ever wasted millions of pounds of taxpayers money. I have an image in my mind of couples up and down the country, where one asks the other, "What should we have for dinner tonight?" and the partner replies, "I think I fancy 600 calories". Public Health England did not specify any particular types of food in their advice; they just want us to consume 600 calories. Eating a delicious meal, with our loved ones, is one of life's greatest pleasures. Public Health England wants to suck all the joy out of it and reduce it to a type of energy accountancy, tinged with guilt. How on earth is anyone supposed to cook and serve a meal of precisely 600 calories per person? Will 600 calories of salmon and broccoli have the same effect on your weight and health as 600 calories of sugar-coated doughnuts? The answer is no and I will soon explain why, but first we need to know what a calorie is. We can't keep talking about calories without knowing what they are.

A calorie is a unit of heat energy. It is defined as *'the amount of energy required to raise the temperature of a gram of water by one degree centigrade at normal atmospheric pressure'*. Carbohydrates and proteins contain 4 calories per gram and fats contain 9 calories per gram. How do we know this? The experiments to determine these values involved placing a gram of each macronutrient into a special container surrounded by water. A stream of oxygen was directed over each sample so it would burn when it was set on fire. When the food samples had burnt out, the heat created had caused a rise in water temperature, which was used to calculate the calorie content of each food type. The calories we see listed on packets of food, and referred to by Public Health England, are kilocalories (Kcal) and one of those is the energy required to raise the temperature of a litre of water by one degree. So, if we manage to calculate and serve 600 calories of food on to our plate, as Public Health England want us to do, will we know how much weight we are going to lose? No, we will not. However, what we will know about our meal is how much it could raise the temperature of a litre of water if we set fire to it.

Public Health England's preoccupation with counting calories is misguided. It implies that the most important thing about our food is how much energy it contains. Instead, we should be thinking about how much nutrition it contains. If our meal has a good supply of all the essential nutrients, amino acids, fatty acids, minerals and vitamins, it is also very likely to contain enough energy. If we think only in terms of energy, we can easily consume 600 calories without getting anywhere near the nutrition we need. For example, 600 calories of cheese omelette has almost every nutrient you need, while 600 calories of an 'energy drink' are entirely devoid of anything resembling an essential nutrient.

Another problem with counting calories is the assumption that all calories are the same. If you are heating water by setting fire to food then all calories have the same effect, but this is not what happens inside our bodies. Our stomachs do not contain a calorie-counting gland. All our bodily functions are controlled by hormones and different types of food produce a different hormonal response. We have known this since the 1950s.

London University's Professor of Medicine, A Kekwick, and research biochemist, G Pawan, published their findings in *The Lancet* on July 28th, 1956. The paper was called: *Calorie intake in relation to body-weight in the obese*. Previous studies, by Lyon and Dunlop in 1932 [2] and Pennington in 1954,[3] had stated that overweight people lost more weight when their diet consisted mainly of fat. Kekwick and Pawan set out to prove this for themselves. They recruited a number of obese people and admitted them to hospital, where their food intake and physical activity could be carefully controlled.

In the first of three experiments, they divided these people into four groups. They all received the same diet consisting of nearly equal proportions of protein, fat and carbohydrate; however, one group ate 2,000 calories of this mixture per day; the second group had 1,500 calories; the third had 1,000 calories; and the fourth group ate only 500. When they were weighed, after a few weeks, the results were as we would expect. The fewer calories people ate, the more weight they lost. A poor scientist, or someone with an agenda, might have stopped there and announced, "Look, I have proved that reducing calories is the way to lose weight". Fortunately, Kekwick and Pawan were good scientists, so they did another experiment.

In their second piece of research, all four groups ate 1,000 calories each day, but the food for the first group was 90% carbohydrate; the second group ate 90% protein; the third group had 90% fat; and the final group ate the original mixed diet. If the number of calories consumed controls weight loss, and it doesn't matter where those calories come from, then all four of these groups should have lost the same amount of weight. The following diagram is taken from the original paper. The results are expressed as weight lost, and therefore, the higher a bar goes up the page the more weight has been lost by that individual. It is clear to see that the people who lost the most weight were eating a diet of 90% fat (the third group from the left). The people who lost the least weight were eating 90% carbohydrate and, despite eating only 1,000 calories per day, some of them managed to put on weight.

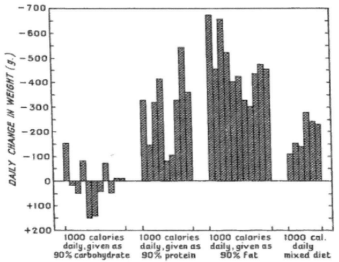

Fig. 7—Daily changes of weight of patients on 1000-calorie diets of different composition (mean of 5-9 days on each diet).

When Kekwick and Pawan saw these results they decided to do a third experiment. They put five people on 2,000 calories per day of the mixed diet and the weight of these subjects remained fairly stable. Then, they raised the calorie intake to 2,600 per day but increased the fat and protein content and reduced the carbohydrate. Four of the five patients lost weight on this diet, despite eating many more calories. This research clearly demonstrated that the type of food we eat is a far more important factor in weight loss than the number of calories we eat. This has been known for over 60 years but few people seem to be aware of it.

The third of these experiments shows that there is no need to reduce calories if we eat a low-carbohydrate, high-fat diet. Significantly, the metabolic problems of an extended, low-calorie diet can be avoided. We do not need to become cold, hungry, lethargic and irritable to lose weight. If we do not need to be hungry, we do not need lots of will power; we just need to eat the right type of food. The correct diet, for weight loss and metabolic health, contains plenty of unprocessed fat and protein, with very little carbohydrate. This is precisely what our ancestors ate during our evolution. It is the opposite of what the NHS and Public Health England have been advising in recent years. The same years that have seen a massive increase in obesity and diabetes.

The details are always the most important part of any argument and it is important to understand what is happening here. If you are thinking that you can simply add lots of fat to your diet and you will lose weight, you are mistaken. It is the reduction in carbohydrate that creates the weight loss. We need to ditch the carbohydrate and replace it with fat.

The NHS does not agree with this. They still cling to the flawed dogma that fat is bad for us and we should replace it with carbohydrate. If you become obese and are unable to lose your excess weight, the NHS policy is to perform bariatric surgery. At a cost of £5,000, they will remove part of your stomach, or put a band around it, to prevent you from eating very much. How can an organisation, dedicated to improving the health of the nation, perform major surgery on a vital organ when there is nothing wrong with it? There is nothing wrong with your stomach; it is the food you are putting into it that is the problem.

Hormones

In the first chapter I said that I would be asking your brain to do something difficult: to unlearn things you had always thought to be true. For many people the idea that 'fat makes you fat' is a deeply ingrained truth which will be hard to dislodge. Vocabulary is part of the problem here. It is an unfortunate coincidence that we use the same word for dietary fat, which is good, as we do for being fat, which is bad, and it appears logical that one would cause the other. But, as I have said before and will say again, the sun appears to travel around the earth although it does not. Fat sounds like it would make us fat but it does not. We become fat because of the action of hormones on our food.

Ghrelin, leptin, insulin and glucagon are all hormones that react to our intake of food. Ghrelin and leptin are both essential for the control of appetite. Ghrelin is produced by the stomach and it tells the brain to create a feeling of hunger when energy is getting low. Its counterpart, leptin, is produced after a meal and it tells the brain to switch off the sense of hunger. As mentioned briefly in Chapter 1, insulin and glucagon control blood sugar levels. Too much sugar in the blood is extremely toxic, so it needs to be kept at a stable level. When blood sugar falls too low, the hormone glucagon prompts the release of glucose from storage, or it instructs the liver to make glucose from proteins. When the sugar level goes too high, insulin is released by the pancreas and it removes excess glucose from the blood by transporting it into cells, where it is used for energy. Insulin also instructs the liver to convert excess glucose into fat and store it in the fat cells. These two pairs of hormones are great examples of the wonderful world of homeostasis.

If this intricate system of controls is so good, how come we eat too much and get fat? The answer, as Kekwick and Pawan demonstrated, is that we eat too much of the wrong things. The National Dietary Guidelines tell us to base our meals on carbohydrates such as bread, potatoes, pasta and rice. All of these foods contain carbohydrate in the form of starch, which is a long chain of glucose molecules joined together. Our digestive enzymes easily slice these glucose molecules off the chain and absorb glucose into the blood stream. This makes the blood sugar level shoot up, which in turn triggers the release of insulin to bring it back to normal. If the cells don't need any more energy and the glycogen store is full, insulin gets the liver to convert the glucose into fat. The blood sugar level now comes down but, if it has spiked high, the pancreas has to produce a lot of insulin and a lot of insulin makes the sugar level fall too low, which triggers a feeling of hunger. You only ate a couple of hours ago but now you feel hungry again. You eat some more carbohydrate and the process repeats itself.

This is known as the blood sugar roller-coaster: blood glucose spikes up; insulin stores the energy as fat; blood sugar comes down too far and you feel hungry. You eat more carbohydrate and blood sugar spikes up again and insulin stores it as fat. This is the reason obese people always keep eating. It is not because they are greedy: it is because they are hungry. They are stuck on an extreme version of the sugar and insulin roller-coaster. The only way to get off is to stop eating food that raises blood sugar. Carbohydrate raises blood sugar and insulin levels further and faster than anything else. Protein raises insulin a little bit but fat hardly moves it all.

Why would our hormones do something so cruel to us? We evolved to be like this and it is not a mistake. The process I have just described is a piece of evolutionary genius. For millions of years our ancestors had no supermarkets, home delivery nor food-filled freezers. Instead, they had to find their food each day. Carbohydrate-rich foods, like berries and fruit, would probably be available only when they were in season, during autumn. Our hormones adapted to this situation by making sure we ate as many berries as we could, during the time they were ripe. We would eat sugary berries and insulin would store the energy as fat. We would feel hungry again and eat more berries until they were all gone. (Bears do this to an amazing extent just before they hibernate.) This built up a good layer of body fat to see us through the winter when we needed more energy to keep warm and there was less food available. It is a brilliant evolutionary adaptation. Well, it was until the 'experts' told us to eat carbohydrate all day, every day and many of us became fat and diabetic.

The way to lose weight, without feeling hungry, is to keep insulin levels low and stable. It has very little to do with calories and a great deal to do with insulin. The way to achieve low insulin is to avoid sugar and keep other carbohydrates to a minimum. Do the opposite of what you are advised and eat a high-fat, medium-protein diet. Above all else, eat real food: food that comes from a farm or a fisherman, not a factory. (I will discuss the perils of processed, food-like substances in a later chapter.) When we eat a high-fat diet, and keep insulin low, we feel full when we have had enough to eat. The hormones, ghrelin and leptin, work as they should do, allowing us to go for long periods of time without thinking about food and never needing to have a snack between meals.

When we switch from a high-carbohydrate, low-fat diet to a low-carbohydrate, high-fat diet, we can feel a bit odd for a few days, as our bodies adjust. This is perfectly normal. We need to start using different hormones and enzymes to power all our energy requirements with fat instead of sugar and it can take a while to make the adjustment. When our bodies become adapted to fat we use molecules called ketones for energy. We are said to be in a state of ketosis and we need to eat a ketogenic diet to maintain ketosis. A very low-carbohydrate, high-fat diet is a ketogenic diet because it triggers the production of ketones.

If all this sounds like a strange fad diet, it is not. We evolved to live this way. The fad diet to worry about is the high-carbohydrate, low-fat diet we have been told to eat since 1983. Babies are born in ketosis to make sure they have plenty of energy to thrive during their first few days of life. A hundred years ago researchers realised that a ketogenic diet was able to prevent seizures in some types of epilepsy.[4] People who eat like this have more mental clarity, less inflammation and better sleep. There are many other health benefits, which I will detail later.

Eat less, move more?
If you are still finding it hard to rewire your brain and remove that Public Health England mantra about needing to 'eat less and move more', I have already demonstrated that eating less is not the answer. What about the 'move more' part? Surely, taking more exercise will use more energy and that will reduce our weight? It sounds logical but logic is unreliable when we don't have all the information we need. Let us take a look at what is going on inside us that makes this logic wrong.

Our bodies have two stores of energy: glycogen and fat. The glycogen store holds about 2,500 calories of readily available glucose and our fat stores can hold an entirely unlimited number of calories. A person who is merely overweight will probably have

100,000 calories stored in their fat cells. When someone, who is not a well-trained athlete, goes running for 20 or 30 minutes, they will use up an extra 300 calories, approximately. If they have insulin in their blood, all of these calories will come from the glycogen store. One of the many functions of insulin is to block access to the fat stores. It does this because a raised insulin level in your blood supply means you have recently eaten carbohydrate and the body wants to burn all that sugar as a priority (because too much sugar is toxic). If you cannot get at your fat stores, you have to use the sugar you have recently consumed. When your run is finished, you will have reduced your glycogen store by 300 calories to 2,200 calories, which will be replenished the next time you eat carbohydrate. Your fat stores will remain completely unaffected by your run, which is very disappointing, because you have to reduce your fat stores to lose weight. The way to lose weight is to reduce carbohydrate intake, which in turn lowers insulin levels. You cannot outrun a bad diet. Exercise bestows a long list of physical and mental health benefits upon us, but helping us to lose significant weight is not one of them.

Banting
Is there any real evidence that a high-fat, low-carbohydrate diet helps people to lose weight? In various places all over the world, where enlightened doctors are advising this approach, thousands of people are losing huge amounts of weight and vastly improving their health. I always like to emphasise that this information is not new, so I will give you an example from the Victorian era. William Banting was an undertaker in London who had become distinctly obese. He hated being so large and complained how difficult it made his daily life. He hated the snide remarks people made about his size and the ailments he was suffering because of it. He sought help from a long list of eminent doctors, who all advised him to 'eat less and move more', which he did to no avail. Eventually, he saw Dr William Harvey who had just returned from Paris where he had attended a conference on diet and diabetes. Dr Harvey decided to try out his new treatment on Banting and advised him to eat meat or fish three times a day, along with any vegetable except for

starchy ones like potato, parsnip and turnip, and to avoid bread, sugar and cakes. The undertaker followed these instructions exactly. He started to lose weight within the first week and continued to do so for months.

Banting referred to his obesity as a 'parasite' invading his body. He was so thrilled to be rid of the parasite that in 1864 he wrote a booklet entitled: *A Letter on Corpulence*.[5] He had 1,000 copies printed at his own expense and gave them away because he saw it as his public duty to pass on the cure for obesity. He and his diet quickly became famous. His booklet eventually sold 63,000 copies and his name became synonymous with dieting. In South Africa, where Professor Tim Noakes is leading the campaign to reduce obesity through low-carbohydrate, high-fat diets, he refers to the process as Banting and people ask each other if they are 'Banting'.

When I was an athlete, I was told to eat a high-carbohydrate diet to make sure I had all the energy I would need. When I was a pharmacist, I was told to advise people to eat a low-fat diet to avoid heart disease. After leaving my career in Pharmacy, I started to question all these things and I began my own research. In a relatively short period of time I have been able to find solid evidence against our national dietary guidelines, against NHS policy and against almost everything Public Health England has to say about food. What is more, the evidence was available long before the dietary guidelines were introduced. Banting wrote his *Letter on Corpulence* more than 150 years ago. Kekwick and Pawan published their results over 60 years ago. If I can find this information from my home computer why can't the 'experts', who are paid to look after our health, find it too?

Summary:
- Weight is controlled by hormones not calories.
- The 'calories in – calories out' theory cannot be successful in the long term because it increases hunger and reduces metabolic rate.

- Weight gain is caused by eating too many carbohydrates, which increase insulin levels. Insulin promotes fat storage and prevents the use of fat for energy.
- The way to lose weight is to restrict carbohydrates and, therefore, reduce insulin. At the same time, we need to maintain calorie intake to prevent a fall in metabolism. The only way to do this is by replacing carbohydrates with healthy fats and proteins. This is the opposite of official advice but it was official advice that caused the obesity epidemic.
- Exercise will not produce weight loss in the presence of too much insulin. We cannot outrun a bad diet.

Chapter 5

SATURATED FAT AND CHOLESTEROL DO NOT CAUSE HEART DISEASE

If we did some research of our own and asked people in the street if it was a good idea to eat butter, cheese and cream instead of bread, potatoes and rice, the vast majority would probably say no. If we asked them why, most of them would say because butter, cheese and cream are full of fat and some would qualify that as saturated fat. If we then asked them what is wrong with saturated fat, some would say, "I don't know, I just know it is bad", while others would say, "it clogs our arteries". We have all been told to avoid saturated fat so often, and for so long, that it seems the majority of people believe it is unhealthy. However, I can guarantee that if we asked 100 of those people to show us the definitive proof that saturated fat is bad, none of them would be able to do so. How can I guarantee this? I can guarantee it because there is no proof and there has never been any proof. Saturated fat is not bad for us and the idea that it clogs our arteries is absurd.

As I explained in Chapter 2, Ancel Keys was responsible for the demonisation of saturated fat because he thought it raised cholesterol, which in turn, caused heart disease. The message to reduce fat, especially saturated fat, was enshrined in the dietary guidelines and repeated so often that everybody thinks it is true. Because of these dietary guidelines, many people are afraid of eating fat. If you are one of those people, I believe it is essential that you overcome this fear and embrace natural dietary fats, which will help you to be healthy and happy. In this chapter, I want to help you to understand the causes of heart disease better than many in the NHS and most GPs. When I was a pharmacist I read, and believed, the professional journals that told me cholesterol was the cause of heart disease and that cholesterol-lowering drugs (statins) would prevent it. Now that I have had time to explore this hypothesis in depth after leaving Pharmacy, I realise it is nonsense and I am annoyed with myself for being so gullible.

The NHS provide a free Health Check for everyone of a certain age and recently I had mine. The nurse and I chatted about how I was feeling as she performed various measurements and tests. My blood pressure (115 / 70) and heart rate (57 and regular) were regarded as ideal. My BMI was also in the correct range. My cholesterol measurements were also considered excellent. Total cholesterol was 4.6; HDL was 1.8 and my total cholesterol to HDL ratio was 2.56. My alcohol intake was not regarded as ideal but I do get plenty of sleep and exercise.

Things got interesting when we started talking about my diet. I was asked about everything except what I eat; I was told what to eat. I was informed I had to avoid saturated fat; only eat lean meat; choose low-fat versions; reduce intake of dairy products; eat lots of carbohydrates and use vegetable oils instead of animal fat. The nurse gave me a verbatim account of the official dietary guidelines. The thing that she didn't know, because I didn't tell her and she didn't ask, is that I drink full-cream milk, I eat full-fat Greek yoghurt, I eat lots of eggs and full-fat cheese. I never cut the fat off meat because it gives the meat more flavour and it is good for me. I never use vegetable oils and cook with either butter, coconut oil or olive oil. I keep my carbohydrate intake low because I don't want to get fat, I don't want diabetes and I don't want Alzheimer's disease.

The thing that bothers me is that she was talking to a man in his sixties with ideal values across a range of health measurements and she never asked me what I eat. There must be thousands of men and women up and down the country having these check-ups and the NHS is completely missing the opportunity to do some research (although it would only be observational). Why don't they want to know what everyone is eating and compare it to each person's blood pressure and cholesterol ratios? I have said it before and I will say it again: the NHS suffers from institutionalised thinking and never questions its own assumptions. How can it ever make a significant difference to the nation's health when it won't examine its own beliefs?

After the check-up, I was sent a Check 4 Life resource pack which contained all my results and some 'helpful information'. On the sheet entitled, 'Cholesterol – The Facts' it correctly states that 'cholesterol is a vital hormone found in every cell of the human body and is produced in the liver and the cells. The human body is very efficient at producing the cholesterol that it needs.' It then goes on to get things wrong by stating that 'excess cholesterol causes a fatty build up on the walls of the arteries, restricting the flow of blood to the heart, brain and other organs'. This is not what happens: it is completely wrong. It is nonsense to suggest that cholesterol sticks to the lining of your arteries like a fat berg in a sewer. Evolution is far too clever for that to happen.

You will have heard of 'good' and 'bad' cholesterol. There is no such thing as bad cholesterol; the concept, however, has been very useful to drug companies because it makes people afraid of cholesterol and, therefore, more likely to take their statin drugs. There is only one cholesterol and it is extremely good. It is a molecule consisting of 27 carbon atoms, 46 hydrogen atoms and one oxygen atom. Like all fats, it does not mix with water and, because our blood is water based, it needs help to travel around the body. The liver makes specialised structures called Lipoproteins. [1] You can think of them like tiny, spherical cargo ships. Their outer surface is not repelled by water so they can travel throughout the blood stream. On the inside they carry cholesterol, triglycerides, which are fats used for energy, and fat soluble vitamins. Depending on their size and content, they are known as High Density Lipoproteins (HDL) or Low Density Lipoproteins (LDL). To be precise, there is a wide range of densities but these two lipoproteins are the ones you hear about most. The things that have been labelled 'good' and 'bad' are, in fact, elaborate structures made of proteins and phospholipids. They are not cholesterol although they carry cholesterol. LDL carries cholesterol (for cell maintenance and repair) and triglycerides (for energy) from the liver to wherever it may be needed in the body, and HDL carries excess cholesterol back to the liver so it can be recycled. It is easier for the liver to recycle precious cholesterol than to make it from scratch.

Heart expert, Dr. Natasha Campbell-McBride, makes the following analogy: "Because cholesterol travels from the liver to damaged cells inside LDL, our 'science' in its wisdom calls LDL bad cholesterol. When the damage heals and the cholesterol is removed, it travels back to the liver in the form of HDL. Because this cholesterol travels away from the damage back to the liver our misguided 'science' calls it good cholesterol. This is like calling an ambulance travelling from the hospital to the patient a bad ambulance and the one travelling from the patient back to the hospital a good ambulance".

What does cause heart disease if it isn't cholesterol? It is true that artery walls can develop thickened areas called plaques and these can grow larger over time. (This is known as atherosclerosis, or hardening of the arteries and often includes deposits of calcium.) The plaques can burst or break free and that can lead to heart attacks and strokes. But what causes the plaques to form in the first place? There is a great deal of debate and it is a complicated story. I will keep the explanation as simple as possible but it is important to realise that heart disease is a process that develops over time. There is no single cause and anything that exacerbates the process will increase the risk of disease. If you want to read about this in depth I recommend *The Great Cholesterol Con* by Doctor Malcolm Kendrick.

Where does plaque occur?
All blood vessels are lined with a special layer of cells called the endothelium. These cells allow all the components of the blood to flow over them, without sticking, because they are flat and smooth. The endothelium produces a substance called Nitric Oxide (NO), which helps to prevent blood from clotting.

Plaques only occur in arteries around the heart, or near it, and never in veins or capillaries. There is one exception to this rule: when a vein is surgically used to create a bypass of a damaged artery, the vein often develops plaque. So, what is it about arteries (and veins used as arteries) that leads to atherosclerosis? Arteries are subjected to much higher blood pressure and more turbulent blood flow than veins. This adds up to a much greater physical stress on the lining of arteries and they are therefore more likely to be damaged. The idea that too much cholesterol in your blood causes plaque cannot explain why plaque only occurs in arteries and not veins. If cholesterol, or saturated fat, clogged our arteries it would surely block our veins and capillaries too but this never happens.

How does plaque occur?

Plaques occur when the endothelium cells are torn, damaged or knocked off. When that happens the blood encounters the layer underneath and this triggers a blood clotting response. A clot forms over the damaged area to protect it and start repair, just as it would when we cut our skin. The big difference is that a scab on the skin falls off when the healing is complete but a scab coming off in an artery would lead to a heart attack or stroke. In your arteries, however, those scabs are absorbed into the tissue and new epithelial cells grow over the top. (I am always amazed how clever our bodies are.)

Normally, the absorbed blood clot is cleared away by the immune system and this process may be happening frequently in healthy people. The problem arises when the same site is damaged again and another blood clot forms. The clear up cells of the immune system (macrophages) can be overloaded and fail to do their job. The blood clot material builds up and the plaque gets bigger.

Why does cholesterol get the blame?

When these plaques were first examined by doctors many years ago, they found significant amounts of cholesterol in them. They assumed that cholesterol was the cause and this assumption is what led to the entire Lipid-Heart Disease Hypothesis and the change in dietary guidelines. Just because cholesterol is found at the site of a problem does not mean it causes the problem. That type of logic would lead us to believe that firefighters cause fires because they are always present when a large building is burning down.

The formation of a clot in a blood vessel is a very complex process, with many different substances involved. As the clot forms it pulls in a lot of the cells circulating in the blood, including red blood cells and lipoproteins. Red blood cell membranes contain a lot of cholesterol and lipoproteins carry cholesterol. Lipoproteins may also travel there specifically to deliver cholesterol to help with the rebuilding process. Thus, a plaque ends up with a lot of cholesterol in it but that does not mean that cholesterol caused it.

What really causes plaque?
There is a list of things that are known to be risk factors for heart disease. It turns out that everything on the list is capable of either damaging the blood vessel lining, or increasing the likelihood of blood clots forming, or reducing the ability of blood clots to be broken down.

The conditions that increase your risk of damage to the artery walls include: high blood pressure; systemic inflammation; high blood sugar/high insulin levels/type 2 diabetes (most diabetics eventually die from heart disease); toxins from cigarette smoke and air pollution; high levels of the stress hormone cortisol; high levels of homocysteine (due to a lack of B vitamins); low levels of vitamin D; drug abuse (especially cocaine); high levels of the clotting agent fibrinogen; and bacterial infection. You will notice that cholesterol is not on the list.

Why do doctors still blame cholesterol?
Anything that disrupts your normal metabolism is a danger to your health and an abnormal lipid profile is no different. Your lipid profile is the ratio of the different types of lipoprotein and the amount of cholesterol and triglyceride they contain. A healthy lipid profile has a high level of HDL particles and a low level of triglycerides. How do you achieve a bad profile? Triglycerides go up far too much when you overload your liver with sugar and carbohydrate. How do you achieve a good profile? A high-fat diet increases HDL and greatly reduces triglycerides.

Another important factor is the size and number of LDL particles. When the liver is overloaded with sugar, which it needs to convert to fat, it produces more triglycerides. When there is more cargo, you need to build more cargo ships. The liver must produce more LDL particles quickly and these are typically very small and dense. In this dietary environment, the LDL particles can become oxidised and it has been shown that oxidised LDL interrupts Nitric Oxide production and directly damages the endothelium cells. This is how cholesterol can be implicated in heart disease, but cholesterol is not the cause. The cause is overloading the liver with too much sugar. Conversely, when we eat a high-fat diet, the liver makes large, fluffy lipoproteins that are more resistant to oxidation. It is not fat that increases your risk of heart disease: it is too much carbohydrate and sugar.

What does cholesterol do?
Cholesterol is vital for human health and we would all die without it. It is an essential component of every cell membrane in the body. The membrane is like the outer wall of a cell and 30% of the membrane is cholesterol.[2] Cholesterol keeps the membrane stable and durable, without being rigid, enabling our cells to change shape and allowing us to move. (Plants don't have cholesterol and their cells are rigid.) It also allows essential nutrients to travel through the membrane and into the cell from the blood stream.

Almost every cell in the body manufactures its own cholesterol, as does the liver. Eating foods high in cholesterol makes no real difference to blood cholesterol because the liver produces less if we eat more and it produces more if we eat less. Consuming foods that are 'low in cholesterol' is a waste of time: you are just giving your liver more work to do.

Cholesterol is necessary to produce our steroid hormones. Steroid hormones help control metabolism, inflammation, immune functions, salt and water balance and all our sexual characteristics and functions. Without cholesterol there would be no reproduction. When we produce vitamin D in our skin it is made from a cholesterol molecule.

There are thousands of miles of nerve fibres in our body which are covered by a myelin sheath. Cholesterol is an essential component of this protective layer. It is so important to the nervous system that 25% of all the cholesterol in our body is found in the brain. Studies in the elderly show that people with higher cholesterol levels live longer than people with low cholesterol and they have far less mental decline and very little memory loss.

Hundreds of millions of years ago evolution developed the cholesterol molecule, which is vital to so many functions in our body. Why would it do that so long ago and then have it start causing heart attacks in 1921? No matter what the 'experts' say, I find it impossible to believe that cholesterol causes heart disease. If you are still finding it hard to unlearn the 'good guy - bad guy' cholesterol story, and you still think cholesterol may be the Grim Reaper's best friend, and you know that statin drugs lower cholesterol to prevent heart attacks, then we should look at some research.

Cholesterol research

In June 2016 the *British Medical Journal Open* published a meta-analysis based on 19 separate studies, which involved over 68,000 participants. (A meta-analysis is a study of the results of a large number of other studies on a particular subject. By combining different studies it is assumed that a true picture will emerge.) The focus of these studies was on the amount of cholesterol inside LDL particles (known as LDL-C), the type of cholesterol we are told is 'bad'. The analysis found that in almost 80% of individuals tested, people with high levels of LDL-C had a lower risk of dying (from any cause) than those with lower levels of cholesterol. Or to put it another way, those who comply with the official guidelines for LDL-C are more likely to die than those who are regarded as "at high risk for heart disease" because they have a raised LDL-C.

In 1985 Dr. George Mann, writing in *Nutrition Today*, said, "A generation of citizens has grown up since the diet-heart hypothesis was launched as official dogma. They have been misled by the greatest scientific deception of our times: the notion that consumption of animal fat causes heart disease".

A major study has shown that women who use statin drugs to lower cholesterol have a much higher risk of developing type 2 diabetes when compared to women who do not. The Women's Health Initiative (WHI) is an American study which recruited 161,800 postmenopausal women, aged 50 to 79 years, at 40 centres across the USA between 1993 and 1998. The latest analysis of data is up to 2005 and includes 153,840 participants, of whom 10,834 were statin users. The average age of all those involved was just over 63 years. The women taking statins had a rate of type 2 diabetes which was 71% higher than those who did not. The increased risk involved all types of statins; there was no difference between the high and low-potency drugs. Cholesterol is a vital molecule for human health and lowering it clearly leads to some major health problems.

There is a group of people with a genetic disorder causing exceptionally high levels of cholesterol to be transported in the blood. It is known as Familial Hypercholesterolemia, which I suggest we refer to as FH. Using the American system of measurement, the medical profession regard 200 mg of cholesterol per 100 ml of blood as the highest safe level. People with FH usually have 350 to 400 mg per 100 ml. If the cholesterol theory is correct, these people must be in greater danger of heart disease than the rest of the population. Statistics show that they do have higher rates of cardiovascular disease. Before you leap up and implore me 'to explain away that one', I need to demonstrate that this is an example of the 'sun goes around the earth thinking' in which the obvious and logical answer is wrong because there is something happening that is hidden.

If high levels of cholesterol cause heart disease, everybody with FH should be affected but they are not. When we compare FH people with heart disease to FH people without heart disease, we find their total cholesterol levels are almost identical and their LDL and HDL are almost identical, but the group with heart disease have higher levels of triglycerides, which we know is a risk factor. The most interesting and decisive measurement is their level of the blood clotting factor prothrombin, which is 2.5 times higher in the group with heart disease than those without it. The genetic variation they possess increases their blood clotting agents, as well as their cholesterol, and, as we discussed above, it is blood clotting that starts the process of swollen artery walls leading to heart attack.

In the *Scandinavian Cardiovascular Journal*, Uffe Ravnskov, MD, PhD wrote: "The cholesterol diet-heart hypothesis is sustained by social, political and financial institutions which have little to do with science or any established success in public-health."

Statin drugs

In 2017 an article was published in the *British Journal of General Practice*. It encouraged doctors to prescribe cholesterol-lowering statin drugs to far more people. It suggested that 11.8 million adults in England, aged 30-84 years, including almost all males over 60 years and all females over 75 years, would be eligible for statin therapy. It claimed that if all these people were treated it would save thousands of lives. When the authorities want to medicate entire groups of people, whether they need it or not, it suggests to me that the interests of the Pharmaceutical industry are more important than the health of individual people.

We are frequently told how useful statins are but when do we hear about the problems they cause? Our bodies have a fantastic system of homoeostasis and if we eat a diet of real, healthy food, our bodily functions remain in harmony. We have a natural level of cholesterol that homoeostasis deems appropriate and to lower it artificially, with drugs, will bring problems. If you have taken statin drugs you may have experienced some of these problems for yourself. The most common side-effect is muscle pain which occasionally leads to muscle damage. This can make exercise very difficult, sometimes impossible, which is ironic when exercise is promoted as an excellent way to reduce heart-disease risk. Statins can also induce liver damage, type 2 diabetes, joint pain, sleep disturbance, headache, dizziness, sexual dysfunction, tinnitus, hair loss and an itchy rash.[3] The worst side-effects, however, are often neurological and include depression and memory loss. Thankfully it is rare, but statins have been linked to Transient Global Amnesia, a terrifying, sudden onset of complete short-term memory loss, which leaves the victim unable to remember where they are or what they are doing.

This happened to Dr. Duane Graveline, a former astronaut, medical researcher and aerospace scientist. His wife found him walking aimlessly and when she spoke to him he did not recognise her. He was rushed to a hospital and six hours later his memory returned. The only medication he was taking was Lipitor, which was the most widely prescribed statin in the world. He stopped taking it, although his doctors refused to believe the cholesterol-lowering drug was the cause. A year later Dr. Graveline was urged to retry half the dose of Lipitor, which he did and six weeks later his entire life was suddenly eradicated from his memory. He had no recall of his children, medical school, years as a flight surgeon nor his time as an astronaut. (If you have been an astronaut, I don't think it is something you are likely to forget.) This episode of amnesia lasted 12 hours.

Dr. Graveline learned of a study, at the University of California, with details of cases just like his own. He set up a website and received thousands of reports from others on statin drugs who had assumed their confusion, disorientation and forgetfulness were caused by getting old. Interestingly, in a recent study that was referred to as a paradox by the medical 'experts', researchers discovered that elderly people with the highest levels of cholesterol had much better recall and memory than people with the lowest levels. [4]

The word *paradox* is often used by obstinate scientists as if it is a 'get-out-of-jail-free' card. When they are presented with evidence that suggests their beliefs and theories are untrue, they call it a paradox, instead of facing up to the reality that they may be wrong. The 'French Paradox' is an excellent example. The people of France consume more saturated fat in their diet than any other European country, yet they have the lowest rates of heart disease in Europe. Scientists who believe saturated fat is bad for us call this a paradox. I call it proof that they are mistaken.

But surely statin drugs reduce the risk of heart attack? Clinical trials of statin drugs have never shown a benefit for women and they have never shown any benefit for men with no previous cardiovascular events. They have shown a small benefit for men who have already suffered a heart attack but around 50 such men would have to take the drugs for five years for one of them to avoid an adverse event. Dr. Kendrick, and others, believe that this small benefit does not come from cholesterol lowering, but is a side effect of statin drugs which produces an increase in nitric oxide, thus reducing blood clotting. The formation of blood clots on damaged artery walls is the start of heart disease.

Another side effect of statins, which can be dangerous, is their potential to increase heart failure. A heart attack is caused by an arterial blockage which prevents blood and oxygen reaching part of the heart. Heart failure is a slow process in which the heart muscles become weaker and, eventually, are unable to pump enough blood around the body to maintain an adequate supply. Muscles need energy which is produced in the mitochondria. A molecule called coenzyme Q10 is an essential component of energy production. Statins work by blocking one of the biochemical steps in the production of cholesterol but this action also blocks the production of coenzyme Q10. Statins are supposed to reduce your chance of a heart attack but they have the potential to increase your chance of heart failure.

If statins are so bad why do we keep seeing stories in the newspapers urging everybody over the age of 50 to take them? These reports always come from the same source, namely the 'Cholesterol Treatment Trialists' Collaboration', known as CTT. This entity is headed by Professor Sir Rory Collins of Oxford University and it holds all the data from drug company trials on statins. He and his co-workers regularly produce scientific papers extolling the virtues of statin treatment. The problem is that he steadfastly refuses to let anybody else see the raw data from these trials.[5] [6] We have to take his word for it. The CTT is closely associated with the Oxford Clinical Trials Service Unit (CTSU) which employs Professor Collins. The CTSU has obtained nearly £300 million in funding from the pharmaceutical industry for running clinical trials on various cholesterol-lowering drugs.

The pharmaceutical industry recently came up with a new class of cholesterol-lowering drugs. They go by the name of PCSK9 inhibitors and they are exceptionally good at taking cholesterol down to extraordinarily low levels. A large scale clinical trial, testing one of these drugs against a placebo, was supposed to run for four years but was stopped after just over two years. Everybody on the drug had greatly reduced cholesterol levels but the number of people suffering heart attacks, and even dying, was slightly higher than the people taking a placebo.[7] Pfizer, the company behind this drug, has now abandoned it. The extreme lowering of cholesterol by this drug showed no health benefits

There is some research I find very worrying. Studies have shown that low cholesterol levels in men, aged 50 or older, are linked to a much higher rate of suicide or violent behaviour.[8] A study in Sweden showed a strong link between low cholesterol levels and violent criminal behaviour. Twenty five per cent of the cholesterol in our bodies is in the brain, and clearly, it is there for a good reason.

Finally, I will quote Dr Malcolm Kendrick, author of *The Cholesterol Con*:

"The dangers of a low cholesterol level were highlighted by a major long-term study of men living in Honolulu: 'Our data agree with previous findings of increased mortality in elderly people with low serum cholesterol, and show that long-term persistence of low cholesterol concentration actually increases the risk of death.'

Somewhat ironically, the danger of a falling cholesterol level was first discovered in the Framingham study: 'There is a direct association between falling cholesterol levels over the first 14 years [of the study] and mortality over the following 18 years.'

It seems almost unbelievable that warnings about the dangers of a high cholesterol level rain down every day, when the reality is that a low cholesterol level is much more dangerous than a high level. Given this, why would anyone want to lower their cholesterol level? On the face of it, it would make more sense to take cholesterol-raising drugs. Especially after the age of 50."

Summary:

- The National Dietary Guidelines were based on the idea that saturated fat raised cholesterol and high cholesterol caused heart disease. When we accept that cholesterol is not the cause of heart disease, the entire premise of the high-carbohydrate, low-fat diet becomes invalid.
- Heart disease is a process which is accelerated by an unhealthy lifestyle and toxic chemicals.
- There is no such thing as bad cholesterol. Cholesterol is made by the liver, and individual cells, because it is essential for human health. Twenty-five per cent of all the cholesterol in our bodies is found in the brain, which is why cholesterol-lowering drugs increase the likelihood of dementia.
- The advice to avoid cholesterol-containing food is completely pointless. The less cholesterol we eat, the more the liver needs to make and vice versa.
- Statin drugs lower the levels of cholesterol in our bodies and that is the reason they cause so many unpleasant side effects. Statins produce a small reduction in heart attacks via the side effect of increasing nitric oxide levels.
- Statins are still heavily promoted as live-saving, wonder drugs but that has far more to do with the billions of dollars of profit they generate, rather than the lives they save.
- Do not fear foods containing saturated fat.

Chapter 6

PURE, WHITE AND DEADLY

When visitors come to your house I expect you probably offer them a cup of tea or coffee. When you ask how they take it, what would you think if one of them said, "I like it with a splash of milk and nine spoons of sugar"? Would you count nine spoons of sugar into the cup or would you ask if that was a joke? Would you just do it or would you refuse to do it because you know it must be bad for them? I hope most people would suggest that nine sugars are just too many.

If, by chance, it was a very warm day and instead of a cup of tea you offered them a cold drink, would you have any qualms about giving them a can of say, Coca-Cola? I only ask because a standard 330ml can of 'Coke' has the equivalent of nine spoons of sugar in it, as do a whole range of other well-known and highly-marketed soft drinks.[1] However, these are not the extreme: they are at the low end of liquid-sugar content. Some of the worst offenders, referred to as 'energy drinks', can contain up to 20 teaspoons of sugar as well as a high dose of caffeine. 'Energy drinks' do not give you energy; they give you tooth decay, heart palpitations, mood swings and diabetes. We have an epidemic of obesity and diabetes and the biggest cause of all this misery is excess sugar. Please don't drink it. Just say no!

In August 2018 the UK Government announced that it was considering banning the sale of energy drinks to anyone under 18 and put the proposal to public consultation. In December of the same year it was announced that 'experts' had advised the Government that there was 'insufficient evidence to warrant a ban on sales of energy drinks to young children'. I think we can speculate that these 'experts' may not have been entirely independent of the sugar industry. The decision is alarming because 97% of experts in children's behaviour, i.e. teachers, who witness the effects of these drinks daily, voted for a ban when they were polled.

The story of 21 year old Vinnie Pyner appeared in a lot of British newspapers during February, 2019. Mr Pyner had started drinking cans of Monster Energy two years earlier and he had become rather fond of them, consuming up to six cans a day. His family's fear that he was overdoing it were confirmed when the young man bit into an apple and all four of his top front teeth snapped.

The title of this chapter, *Pure, white and deadly*, is my homage to Professor John Yudkin who wrote a book with this title in 1972. I mentioned him in Chapter 2, when I explained how Ancel Keys had destroyed the careers of anyone who disagreed with his theory that saturated fat caused heart disease. Yudkin was convinced that fat was not the problem: the problem was sugar. In his book he wrote, "If only a small fraction of what we know about the effects of sugar were to be revealed in relation to any other material used as a food additive, that material would promptly be banned." He was sure that the over-consumption of sugar was the root cause of a great many modern, lifestyle diseases.

Applying logical thought, he said that while humans have always been carnivorous, carbohydrates only became a major component of our diet 10,000 years ago with the advent of mass agriculture. Sugar has been part of western diets for only about 300 to 500 years, which in evolutionary terms is moments ago. Saturated fats, by contrast, are so completely interwoven with our evolution that they are abundantly present in breast milk. To Yudkin's thinking, it seemed much more likely to be the recent innovation of sugar that was making us ill, rather than the prehistoric staple of saturated fat. In this chapter, I will explain how sugar is the root cause of so much modern disease.

Sugar is the generic name for all sweet-tasting, soluble carbohydrates. The various types of sugar are derived from different sources. Simple sugars are called monosaccharides and include glucose (also known as dextrose), fructose, and galactose. Table sugar, or granulated sugar, refers to sucrose, which is a disaccharide consisting of a glucose molecule attached to a fructose molecule. In the body, sucrose is split into fructose and glucose. When we talk about sugar we usually mean table sugar but when we talk about blood sugar we really mean blood glucose.

Diabetes

There are about 4 million people in the UK who have been diagnosed with type 2 diabetes and there are probably millions more who are not yet diagnosed, or who have pre-diabetes and will soon have the full disease. (This section is about type 2 diabetes and when I write 'diabetes', I am only talking about type 2 diabetes.) It has become so common, I worry that some people may be slightly too relaxed about it but it is an awful disease and nobody should be blasé. Most people would say that diabetes is too much glucose in the bloodstream. It is true that diabetics have too much sugar in their blood but that is not really the disease: it is a symptom of the disease. The real disease is Insulin Resistance, which can also be referred to as Carbohydrate Intolerance. It can be a truly awful disease.

If you have diabetes it will degrade your blood vessels. The tiny capillaries in your kidneys and the retina of your eyes can become so damaged that you need kidney dialysis and may go blind. Diabetes also greatly increases the risk of heart disease and stroke and this is the major cause of death in diabetic people. Some of your nerve fibres can be damaged causing neuropathic pain: a nagging pain that normal pain killers do not control.

Men can suffer from erectile dysfunction and women can suffer complications in pregnancy. Alzheimer's disease is now being referred to as type 3 diabetes because research has shown a huge link with insulin resistance and various forms of dementia and cognitive decline.[2] The damaged blood vessels in your legs reduce the blood flow to your feet and this leads to ulcers that will not heal. These ulcers can develop gangrene and then you will have to have your toes, feet or legs amputated. In England alone, 120 diabetics have part of a limb amputated every single week. I think this is worth repeating: over 6,000 people in England and millions around the world have part of a limb amputated every year because they eat too much carbohydrate. If you are still not convinced how awful diabetes is, you could type "diabetic amputations" into a search engine and then press images. I warn you that it is not for the squeamish.

A healthy adult circulation contains about 10 pints of blood with one teaspoon (or 5 grams) of glucose dissolved in it. The level of glucose is very strictly controlled. When it falls too low, the hormone glucagon is released and glucagon brings glucose out of storage and into the blood. If the level rises too high, the hormone insulin is released and insulin transports glucose out of the blood and into the cells. If the cells don't need any more glucose and the storage area is full, insulin gets the liver to convert the extra glucose into fat and stores it in the fat cells.

Obesity is closely linked to diabetes because of insulin: if insulin did not convert excess glucose to fat and store it away, you would become diabetic whenever you ate too much starchy food. (Starch is just a lot of glucose molecules joined together.) Putting on weight is the body's way of avoiding diabetes. Eventually though, the body cannot cope anymore and the system breaks down and blood sugar goes up. A lot of different factors, including genetics, are involved in deciding who this happens to and when it happens. Obesity and diabetes are linked because they are both symptoms of insulin resistance. Obesity doesn't cause diabetes: they are both caused by too much sugar.

Diabetes has a genetic component but genetics does not cause it. The nuance is important. If 100 people are fed a diet very high in refined carbohydrates and sugar, they will all put on weight but only some of them will develop diabetes. The people who are genetically predisposed to it will become insulin resistant on such a diet, while other people's genes may protect them from the disease. However, genetics did not make them ill: too much sugar made them ill. If these same 100 people had been fed a very low carbohydrate diet instead, none of them would have become diabetic. The wrong diet creates diabetes; genetics decides who succumbs to it.

What causes insulin resistance? Insulin does. The first time you drink alcohol it takes very little for you to feel tipsy. When you have been drinking for years, it takes a lot more alcohol to have the same effect because your body has become resistant to it. As we have discussed in other chapters, carbohydrates are converted to glucose which raises the blood sugar and increases insulin production. Over the years an excess of insulin in the blood makes your cells resistant to it, and then it cannot do its job. Blood sugar goes up, which stimulates more insulin production, leading to more resistance, and suddenly, you have diabetes.

These are some of the common symptoms of diabetes: increased thirst; frequent urination; dry mouth; unexplained weight loss; feeling tired and weak; blurred vision with headaches; and recurrent infections, especially thrush. If you go to your doctor with any of these symptoms you will be given some tests, and if you have high levels of blood glucose you will be told that you have type 2 diabetes. It is very likely that you will also be told that diabetes is a progressive, incurable disease. You will be given medication which either increases sensitivity to insulin or increases insulin production. You will also be told to control your diet. Unfortunately, the dietary advice you are likely to get will make your diabetes worse. The standard advice is to eat plenty of fruit, vegetables and whole grains and to reduce the amount of fat you eat, in a mistaken attempt to lose weight. If you want to avoid diabetes, or make it go away if you already have it, you should completely ignore the official dietary advice.

Diabetes is a disease of too much insulin but when the tablets no longer work they will inject you with insulin. The only food group that does not stimulate insulin is fat and they want you to avoid it. Fruit and whole grains have high levels of carbohydrate which raise your blood sugar and insulin. If you follow the official advice, you will discover that what they told you told is true: diabetes is progressive and incurable. If you ignore the official advice and eat a low-carbohydrate, high-fat (LCHF) diet, you will avoid diabetes and quite probably reverse it if you already have it. **Please note,** if you are taking medication for diabetes and you change to a low-carbohydrate, high-fat diet you must tell your doctor and monitor your blood very closely because your sugar levels will fall and the medication may precipitate a hypo. Some people may suggest that I am promoting a dangerous, newfangled fad diet. The truth is that people have known how to deal with diabetes for a long time. Unfortunately, we have forgotten the simple approach of diet and replaced it with medication, which of course is very profitable for drug companies.

Diabetic Cookery, Recipes and Menus, a book by Rebecca Oppenheimer, was published in 1917. The book gives detailed advice on what to eat and what to avoid for people with diabetes. All the information must have come from experience and observation because the hormone insulin was not discovered until four years later, in 1921. We live in the era of the 'expert' and we are guided constantly by official advice which, in my opinion, diminishes our ability to trust our instincts and act upon our experiences, unless they are validated by a higher authority. It is depressing to realise we were better able to advise type 2 diabetics 100 years ago. On page 12 of the book there is a list of *"especially valuable foods, because of their great nutritive qualities"* and it includes butter, olive oil, cream, stilton, cheddar, brie, bacon, ham, pork, beef, mutton, goose, mackerel, salmon, caviar and eggs. These are all high in fat and protein and very low in carbohydrate.

On the following page, Rebecca Oppenheimer has a list of foods which are strictly forbidden. It includes sugar, puddings, flour, bread, biscuits, oatmeal, macaroni, all sweet and dried fruits, honey, syrups, beer and all farinaceous foods. Farinaceous is a word we do not use any more but it means starchy foods, especially roots and tubers. Everything on the forbidden list is a carbohydrate.

Dr. Jason Fung is a nephrologist, a kidney specialist, working in Toronto, Canada. He sees diabetic patients with kidney damage every day but instead of just putting them on dialysis, he reverses their diabetes with intensive, dietary management and intermittent fasting. He uses a low-carbohydrate, high-fat diet coupled with the omission of some meals, to reduce their insulin levels and put their diabetes into remission. There are many examples of success on his website, idmprogram.com

Dr. David Unwin, a GP in Southport, treats diabetics with a low-carbohydrate diet. His surgery has the most successful treatment regime of any in the UK. He achieves reversal of the disease and drug-free continuation in 40% of his patients, despite having been told as a student that diabetes is progressive and incurable. He has reduced spending on diabetes care in his surgery by £40,000 per year because his approach reduces, or eliminates, the need for drugs and insulin. Imagine how much money the NHS could save if all doctors realised that diabetes is caused by diet and can be reversed by diet. In November 2018 the NHS announced they were going to tackle diabetes by allowing doctors to prescribe special milkshakes containing only 800 calories. Patients would be required to have no more than three per day and would stay on this protocol for three months. The NHS said the weight loss this would produce had been shown to reverse diabetes in half of the people who had been tested. How can the NHS be so foolish? Dr. Unwin has shown them how to deal with diabetes at no cost to the health service, but instead they have decided to buy milkshakes for people. These shakes are ultra-processed, chemical soups. The main ingredients are fat-free-milk protein, sugar and canola oil. This is the sort of junk that made people ill in the first place. The NHS appear to be unaware that a starvation level of calories, whilst ensuring some weight loss, also causes muscle loss and serious psychological problems, as well as rebound weight gain after returning to 'normal' eating.

Tooth decay

There is an epidemic of tooth decay in Britain. Dental surgeons in the NHS are performing record numbers of operations to pull out rotten teeth in children. During a 12 month period spanning 2016 and 2017, hospitals extracted multiple teeth from children and teenagers in England a total of 42,911 times. That is a 17% increase on the 36,833 procedures carried out by surgical teams in 2012-13. The figures were bad back then but they are getting worse.

The cause of all this pain, misery and expense is sugar, especially sugar-sweetened drinks. Like the rest of our digestive system, our mouths contain a great many bacteria and these bacteria like nothing more than to have all our teeth coated in sticky sugar. Bacteria possess enzymes that convert sugar into an acid, which burns a hole through the tough enamel protecting all our teeth. Once they get through the enamel, they can rot the teeth from the inside. Eating sugary sweets and drinking sugar-laden, fizzy drinks applies sugar onto all the teeth, which is just what those bacteria want.

Our teeth are the hardest and toughest component of the entire digestive tract. If sugar can destroy them, imagine what it may be doing to the rest of our insides? The way to prevent tooth decay is to avoid sugar.

Cancer

Otto Warburg was a German doctor who lived from 1883 to 1970. He won the Nobel prize for Physiology in 1931 for his work on energy production in the mitochondria of our cells. He demonstrated that normal cells use oxygen to extract energy from a ketone molecule called pyruvate but cancer cells are unable to do this. They rely on the fermentation of glucose for energy. Warburg suggested that cancer cells could be defeated by starving them of glucose, which is their only source of energy. More recently, specialists in cancer have suggested that this is a 'chicken and egg' situation. They believe cancers are caused by genetic mutations, and the mutations cause the change in the way cancer cells use energy.

Nowadays, we know that people with obesity and diabetes are considerably more likely to develop cancer. Why would obese people be more likely to have random mutations in the genes which control energy production than a slim person? Obesity and diabetes are caused by too much carbohydrate and sugar and Warburg demonstrated that cancer needs a ready supply of sugar to thrive. Research has shown that there is a very strong increase in the risk of cancer for people with permanently elevated blood sugar whether they are obese or slim.[3] It is the sugar level, not necessarily your weight, that is the problem.

Cancer cells grow and multiply rapidly and it is, therefore, important to reduce anything that stimulates cell growth. Insulin is a growth promoter and it is elevated when we eat too much sugar. Being overweight is a risk in itself because excessive adipose tissue, which is the medical name for fat cells, causes an increase in the levels of some hormones, particularly oestrogen, and this too is a growth promoter. To reduce the risk of cancer, we need to do the same thing that reduces the risk of diabetes, tooth decay and obesity. We need to do the opposite of the dietary guidelines and eat a low-carbohydrate, high-fat diet.

Alzheimer's disease

Along with other forms of dementia, Alzheimer's disease is becoming more common. It is an awful disease, as anyone whose loved ones suffer from it will testify. It can begin with forgetfulness but progress to the point of almost total amnesia, where people do not know who their own children are. Sufferers are typically unable to remember what happened a few minutes ago but are able to tell stories from the distant past. Sadly, they often tell the same stories over and over again because they cannot remember having just told them. In the latter stages of the disease, when too many brain cells have died, the symptoms can include: insomnia; inability to swallow; mood changes including depression; incontinence; hallucinations and delusions.

The pharmaceutical industry has spent billions of pounds on research for a drug to treat Alzheimer's disease. The search has been in vain. Their attempts to find a cure have been the most expensive failure in the entire history of medical research. They have been looking for a way to eliminate tangled proteins, called amyloid plaque, that appear in the brains of those with the disease. They should have been looking for the root cause.

Scientists are beginning to realise that Alzheimer's disease is another manifestation of insulin resistance and they have started to call it Type 3 Diabetes. Alzheimer's disease often begins with Vascular Dementia, which as its name suggests, is deterioration of brain tissue caused by damaged blood vessels. As we have discovered, too much sugar leading to insulin resistance causes damage to blood vessels in the retina of the eye, to the kidneys and to the feet. Why wouldn't it cause blood vessel damage in the brain? Eating a high-carbohydrate, low-fat diet increases your chance of dementia. People with type 2 diabetes have a higher incidence of Alzheimer's disease than people with normal blood sugar.

Epilepsy and other brain disorders

Epilepsy is a disease involving repeated seizures or fits. These are sudden bursts of electrical activity in the brain, temporarily altering how it works. Seizures can affect people in different ways depending on which part of the brain is involved. Some seizures cause the body to jerk and shake, whilst others cause problems like loss of awareness or unusual sensations. They typically pass in a few seconds or minutes. The standard treatment is to take drugs to prevent or reduce the seizures. Patients often have to try several different medicines to discover the one that works best for them. Many of these drugs have some unpleasant side effects and sometimes they just do not work at all.

Almost 100 years ago, in 1923, Dr. Russell Wilder discovered that some people, with hard-to-control epilepsy, were able to reduce, and in some cases eliminate, their seizures by eating a ketogenic diet. As described earlier, a ketogenic diet is sufficiently low in carbohydrate and high in fat that the body no longer relies on glucose for energy, but uses molecules called ketones instead. Ketones are produced by the liver from the fat we eat or have stored. It appears that ketones are able to reduce the excitability of brain cells that trigger epileptic seizures. Also, ketones produce energy without creating the damage-causing 'reactive oxygen species' that are typical of glucose metabolism. Ketones produce energy in the mitochondria of our cells without inflammation and oxidative stress.

Jim Abrahams is the American film director of comedies like *Airplane* and *Naked Gun*. His son, Charlie, developed severe epilepsy when he was almost a year old. The little boy was having a hundred seizures a day. The first drug he was given did not help his fits but did cause side effects. Subsequent drugs were no better. Specialists carried out brain surgery but that did not work either. Jim Abrahams became desperate and studied everything he could find on the treatment of epilepsy. Eventually, he stumbled upon a book that recommended the ketogenic diet. Against the advice of his neurologist, he took Charlie to a ketogenic specialist at John Hopkins University. The Abrahams family were taught how to create a diet for their little boy consisting of 90% fat, 6% protein and 4% carbohydrate. Along with the new diet, they stopped all medication and within 48 hours his seizures had ceased. Charlie is now in his twenties with no sign of epilepsy.

The Abrahams family were delighted to have Charlie's health restored but then they became angry because they had never been told about this therapy. They had stumbled upon it themselves, despite its well documented longevity and success. In response, they created the Charlie Foundation to promote the benefits of ketogenic therapy in the treatment of epilepsy.

A paper published in *Frontiers in Pharmacology,* in 2012, by Carl Stafstrom, University of Wisconsin, looked at the effects of a ketogenic diet on a whole range of neurological disorders. Several diseases causing debilitating physical symptoms are all a consequence of the degeneration, or even the death, of certain brain cells. We have already mentioned epilepsy and Alzheimer's disease but some studies have suggested it is possible that Parkinson's disease, motor neurone disease, autism, depression, bipolar disorder and migraine could all be helped with a ketogenic diet. These dreadful ailments display a wide variety of symptoms but they all stem from brain cells that do not function properly and we know that ketones help brain cells to stabilise.

Unfortunately, there will be very little scientific research done on diet for all these brain dysfunctions. Clinical trials cost a lot of money and drug companies will never fund research that demonstrates there is no need for their medications. According to a video on the Charlie Foundation website (charliefoundation.org), the reason Jim Abrahams was not told about the ketogenic diet is because pharmaceutical companies persuade doctors of the benefits of their drugs above all else. If it is discovered that all these brain diseases can be improved by changing to a diet containing meat, eggs, butter and cream, the drug companies will lose a great deal of profit.

Aggression in children

According to research carried out by Bar Ilan University in Israel, there is a strong and consistent relationship between a child's sugar consumption and violent behaviour. The researchers used data from a study called *Health Behaviour in School-Aged Children*, carried out by the University of St Andrews and the World Health Organisation, in 2013-14. In the UK, they found that children who consume a lot of sweets and energy drinks are 89% more likely to smoke and 72% more likely to drink alcohol as they get older. They are more than twice as likely to get into fights and also likely to be a bully.

Heart disease

Apart from all the causes of heart disease listed in Chapter 4, there are other cardiac problems caused by too much sugar. The surface of each endothelium cell, which line the arteries, is covered by a great many very fine hairs called the glycocalyx. These hairs protect the underlying endothelium from damage, promote nitric oxide release, prevent blood clotting and prevent the adhesion of white blood cells and platelets. Too much sugar in the blood causes severe damage to this protective layer, which increases the chance of blood clot formation.

The main arteries around the heart do not get their blood supply from the blood rushing through them: it moves too quickly to allow proper absorption of nutrients and oxygen. Instead, these vessels have their own blood supply via tiny capillaries on the outside of the artery known as the vasa vasorum. Too much sugar in the blood causes damage to the tiniest of capillaries leading to insufficient oxygen getting to the artery which, in turn, increases the risk of endothelial damage.

Acne

Acne usually occurs in teenagers but can affect adults too. It is cruel that unsightly acne erupts at the stage in life when we are most self-conscious. It is often thought to be caused by the changing hormones of puberty and while they surely have an effect, it does not explain acne in adults. Our old friend insulin stimulates the production of androgen hormones. Androgens are male hormones but they are present in both men and women. They can contribute to acne by overstimulating the oil glands and altering the development of skin cells that line hair follicles in the skin.

Infertility and PCOS

Infertility is a frustrating and distressing condition for young couples who are desperate to start a family. The typical solution to this problem, often only reached after months of intrusive tests, is a course of IVF (in vitro fertilisation) at a cost of £5,000 per cycle. Couples often need up to three cycles to achieve success.

PCOS stands for polycystic ovarian syndrome. It is an increasing problem in the UK and around the world, with one in every five women thought to be affected by it. The symptoms include: irregular periods or no periods at all; infertility; excessive hair growth on the face, back, chest or buttocks; simultaneous hair loss from the head; weight-gain; and oily skin or acne. A hairy chest and bald head are typical male characteristics caused by male sex hormones. Infertile women have androgen levels that are too high for their ovaries to work as they should

Dr. Michael D. Fox is Medical Director at Jacksonville Center for Reproductive Medicine. His days are spent helping women to become more fertile. He tells them to "Eliminate carbohydrate from your diet and add real butter, whipping cream, hard cheeses, homemade mayonnaise, pork and olive oil."

In the UK, Dr. Gillian Lockwood, executive director of fertility group IVI, said she advises all patients to cut their carbohydrate intake, amid a growing body of evidence linking such foods to impaired fertility.

All of these diseases and health problems are not only costing the National Health Service a fortune, whilst putting medical staff under terrible pressure, but above all causing needless suffering to thousands of people. Tragically they have all been created, or made worse, by that ill-conceived idea to reduce dietary fat and increase carbohydrate.

Summary:

- For millions of years our ancestors ate very little sugar but now we consume huge quantities of it. Too much sugar in the blood stream is toxic and to counteract this the body produces insulin to transport the excess sugar into the cells or turn it into fat.
- Repeated spikes of sugar, followed by insulin, lead to excessive fat storage and insulin resistance. This causes blood sugar levels to rise, leading to type 2 diabetes. If allowed to progress, diabetes will cause blindness, kidney failure, dementia, amputations and death from heart disease.
- Too much sugar causes tooth decay, acne, mood swings, infertility and aggression.
- Cancer cells need a supply of sugar to thrive and a very low-carbohydrate, or ketogenic, diet can inhibit cancer growth.
- Recent research is implicating sugar and starchy carbohydrates in the tragic increase in brain disorders like Alzheimer's disease, epilepsy, dementia, migraine, Parkinson's disease and bipolar disorder.
- Too much sugar is one of the causes of heart disease.

Chapter 7

PURE, WHITE AND HEALTHY

The Book of Revelations warns us about the arrival of the four Horsemen of the Apocalypse: Pestilence, Warfare, Famine and Death. It is not a book I recommend if you want to cheer yourself up. When it was written, over 2000 years ago, riding a horse was the fastest and most impressive mode of transport available. If Revelations was written now, perhaps they would be the four intercontinental, nuclear missiles of the Apocalypse, but this is a book about health and happiness so we will avoid that subject.

There is, it appears, a new version of this story but it only has three horsemen and they are called Sugar, Salt and Fat. We are constantly told to avoid these three substances because we are led to believe they will bring about an apocalypse for our health. It is almost impossible to hear a dietician or nutritionist interviewed on television without blaming this evil gang of three for all our ailments. I realise I am mixing up my references but do you remember the song by Meatloaf called *Two out of three ain't bad?* Perhaps it was acceptable to get two things right out of three in his relationship, but in official, dietary advice we should expect three out of three to be correct. It is very disappointing, therefore, to realise the experts have scored one out of three. They are correct about sugar but salt and fat are vital for our health and to put them together with sugar is illogical, unscientific and incorrect.

Salt, sodium chloride, is vilified because it is believed to raise blood pressure and high blood pressure is one of the risk factors for heart disease. The evidence against salt comes from a study in the 1970s by Lewis Dahl.[1] He raised the blood pressure in laboratory rats by feeding them extra salt and thus claimed he had proved that salt increases the risk of heart attacks and strokes. Healthcare experts started telling everyone to cut back on salt consumption and have continued to do so ever since. However, when we look closely at Dahl's research, we discover that he was feeding the rats the human equivalent of 500 grams per day, which is 50 times the normal intake. We are not rats and nobody eats that much salt. It is a wonder those rats survived long enough to have their blood pressure taken.

In 1988 there was a study on humans called Intersalt. It was an international study of people from 52 different parts of the world. It measured their excretion of sodium and compared that to their blood pressure. The level of sodium we excrete is linked to the amount of salt we consume. The results showed that a higher intake of salt was associated with higher blood pressure. As we already know, higher blood pressure is associated with an increased risk of heart disease, and therefore, we should all slash our salt intake to avoid a lethal heart attack. In the UK, we are advised to eat no more than 6 grams of salt per day. This is equivalent to one teaspoonful and contains 2.4 grams of sodium. The NHS website states that we all eat too much salt and lists many common foods that contain salt.

Is anything in human nutrition ever as simple as this? No, it is not. We have already seen how the vital nutrient cholesterol was wrongly blamed for heart disease, causing an array of side effects in people taking statin drugs. Our bodies function well because of the elaborate balance that homeostasis exerts. When we blame, and restrict, one component of the system for a particular disease, we can throw the entire system out of balance, which inevitably makes our overall health worse not better.

The authorities blithely tell us to eat no more than 6 grams of salt per day but how are we supposed to measure that? How can we possibly know how much sodium chloride is in all the different things we eat? If we had nothing better to do, we could measure the salt we sprinkle on our food but processed food has added salt and many unprocessed foods have naturally occurring salt. We are being asked to do something which is practically impossible and the outcome is that we develop a fear of salt and so avoid it. The experts have managed to make us fear the consumption of a nutrient that is vital for life.

The reduction in blood pressure observed in the Intersalt study was small. A 50% reduction in salt intake produced a drop in blood pressure of 2 millimetres of mercury. This means if your systolic pressure was 140, it would fall to 138 if you cut out half of your salt intake. How many lives is this going to save? A major problem with the results of the study is the inclusion of 'outliers'. These are measurements that are a long way away from the rest of the results. Four indigenous populations from Brazil, Papua New Guinea and two from Kenya were included and they all had very low salt intake and low blood pressure. Their results were so far outside the other readings that they skewed the average of all the others. These people lived a hunter-gatherer lifestyle and ate no processed food at all. Their lives, and their genetics, are so different to the average modern-day westerner that they should never have been included. When those four readings are taken out of the study, there is no clear evidence that salt reduction lowers blood pressure; therefore, the entire premise of reducing salt to lower the risk of heart disease has no reliable science behind it.

Large scale surveys of American dietary habits are carried out occasionally by a group called The National Health and Nutrition Examination Survey (NHANES). They found that people eating the least salt died at a rate that was 18% higher than those eating the most salt.[2] Another of their surveys showed that a low-salt diet was associated with a 15.4% increased risk of death. Other trials found an increased risk of heart attacks among hypertensive patients eating a low salt diet. Patients with hypertension (high blood pressure) are the very people doctors had been advising to cut back on salt.

Research often concentrates on the effect of sodium but salt is half sodium and half chloride. Very little work has been done on the impact of chloride levels and health. The studies that have been done, however, agree that the lower the level of chloride in the blood, the higher the risk of an early death.

As with everything else in our bodies, the details are crucial. The broad brush, one-size-fits-all approach is never going to provide the best advice. In his book, *The Salt Fix,* Doctor James DiNicolantonio explains that 20% of the population are salt sensitive and they tend to have increasing blood pressure with a high salt intake. The other 80% of people show insignificant changes in blood pressure with more salt. The recommendation to reduce salt intake may be correct for people who are salt sensitive, or who have kidney disease; however, for everybody else it is likely to do more harm than good.

What does history have to say about salt?
Our blood is a salt solution with a similar concentration to that of sea water. Millions of years ago life began in the sea and it is believed that the salty blood of all animals is a carry-over from that distant time. For thousands of years salt has been a substance of great importance and value. In his book, *A World History of Salt*, Mark Kurlansky explains: "Salt is so common, so easy to obtain, and so inexpensive that we have forgotten that from the beginning of civilisation until about 100 years ago, salt was one of the most sought-after commodities in human history."

Ancient Greeks, Egyptians and Romans used salt in offerings to their gods. Some Muslims believe that salt protects them from the 'evil eye'. During the Middle Ages spilling salt was considered an omen of misfortune, and the spiller had to throw a pinch over his left shoulder to cast out the devil.

As civilisations grew and agriculture spread across the globe, salt became one of the first commodities to be traded internationally. The production of salt was one of the world's first industries, and considerable effort and expense was committed to obtaining it. Trade routes for salt spread as far and wide as Africa, Asia, the Middle East, and Europe. Salt was often used as money, and was coveted, hoarded, searched for, traded, and even fought over.

The importance of salt has even become part of our language as a metaphor for goodness. People who work hard are known to be 'worth their salt', and the best of people are known as 'the salt of the earth'. The word 'salt' has its origins in the Latin 'sal' and some modern words are derived from this. For example, *salubrious* means health giving and *salary* comes from the money given to Roman soldiers to buy salt. Even the Roman goddess of health and prosperity was called Salus.

Pliny the Younger was a Roman author and prolific letter writer 2,000 years ago. Among his wide-ranging topics were some words on salt. He recommended a little salt under the tongue every morning to prevent tooth decay and also stated, 'sweet foods make us fat, while salt foods make us thin'. He was correct with all these observations. Salt is an antibacterial agent that is still used as a gargle and mouthwash and we now know that sugar makes us fat. Observation was the only research tool available to people thousands of years ago: it was important to them and they paid attention to it. I believe we can all be extremely confident that, if people with a high salt intake were dying sooner than people with a low intake, somebody across all those hundreds of years would have noticed.

In *The Salt Fix,* DiNicolantonio explains that the main method of preserving food for 8,000 years has been to cover it in salt. He has information to suggest that in the 1500s, people across Europe were consuming about 40 grams of salt per day and, at times in the 1700s, it reached as much as 70 grams per day. Throughout human history we ate large amounts of salt, and it is only since the arrival of the 'nutritional expert' that we have slashed our daily intake to 6 grams or less.

Facts about salt
Salt is required not only to protect us from becoming overly dehydrated but is also essential for the maintenance of a high blood volume, ensuring each cell in our body receives the oxygen and nutrients it needs. This high blood volume does not cause excessive blood pressure because salt helps to relax and dilate the blood vessels. Salt also maintains the volume of liquid that exists between all our cells: the extracellular fluid. This salty bath around each cell increases the metabolic rate of the cell, leading to more heat and energy production. Most of the salt in our blood is disassociated, which means it is split into sodium ions and chloride ions. These ions play a vital role in the nervous system by helping nerve signals to travel along nerve fibres. These nerve impulses are

essential for movement and to keep our hearts beating. Chloride ions are used to make the hydrochloric acid in our stomachs that is so vital to digestion, and also for the destruction of harmful bacteria we may have swallowed.

Salt can help us to sleep better, and lower anxiety, because it reduces the effect of the stress hormones cortisol and adrenaline.[3] If you wake up in the middle of the night with your heart racing, try taking some salt washed down with water. Excess salt is stored in our bones, along with other minerals, as well as in the skin. Salt in the skin acts as a natural antiseptic helping to reduce the chance of a cut becoming infected.

Salt is a vital nutrient that we must eat and normal blood contains about 6.7 grams of it. The NHS recommends that we restrict our intake to less than 6 grams per day. Our blood also contains about 5 grams of sugar, which is a substance we do not need to eat at all, but the NHS recommends that we eat approximately 300 grams of sugar-forming carbohydrate every day. Official advice is to restrict something we need and to eat large amounts of something we do not need. How does that make sense?

We are also advised to drink anything from two to four litres of water every day and to drink before we feel thirsty. Professor Tim Noakes is a world-leading physiologist and in his book, *Waterlogged,* he explains why this notion is harmful. The original research that promoted this idea was funded by the American sports-drinks company, Gatorade. They, and other similar organisations, have made a lot of money out of this 'advice'. Noakes systematically dismantles all the arguments used to promote over-hydration and advises everybody to remember that evolution gave us a fail-safe mechanism to regulate water intake: thirst. If we feel thirsty we should drink; if we are not thirsty, there is no need to drink. The problem with Noakes' advice is that global corporations are not going to make a fortune out of it.

What happens if we follow the recommendations to restrict salt and combine that with the notion, funded by the drinks industry, of drinking four litres of water every day? Excessive water produces excessive urine. The kidneys filter this extra fluid out of the body and salt goes along with it. The kidneys expend a lot of energy reabsorbing salt but they never reabsorb all of it and the more water we drink, the more salt we lose. We also lose salt when we sweat. If we do not eat enough salt to replace these losses we become deficient, and if we keep drinking we develop a condition called hyponatraemia, which is the medical name for very low levels of sodium in the blood.

Like most things in the body, hyponatraemia occurs on a sliding scale. Mild hyponatraemia is common in the elderly and leads to abnormalities with walking and movement, leading to an increased risk of falls and fractures. It can also weaken bone structure, making fractures more likely to occur after a fall. Mild hyponatraemia is known to cause problems with cognition, short-term memory loss, disorientation, confusion, depression and difficulty with concentration. Sudden hyponatraemia can result in life-threatening complications, as a result of cerebral oedema (swelling of the brain), which in turn leads to coma and fits.[4] This can be fatal. Marathon runners, who drank lots of water instead of electrolyte-replacement drinks, have died at or near the end of their 26-mile run from sudden hyponatraemia.

There are no recorded deaths from dehydration in long-distance runners. However, if you are severely dehydrated and taken to hospital, you will be put on a saline drip. It is quite common to have 2 litres of salt solution infused into your vein in such circumstances. Saline is a solution of 0.9% sodium chloride, which means that 2 litres contains 18 grams of salt. The health authorities tell us to restrict salt intake to 6 grams or less per day but they will happily inject 18 grams of it into your veins to save your life when you are dehydrated.

Unintended consequences
As we know, insulin is the hormone that controls blood sugar levels, but insulin is a master hormone with many roles in the body. When salt levels are low and the kidneys are trying hard to retain it, insulin is recruited to help with the reabsorption of sodium. When our salt levels remain low, we have elevated insulin, which increases the chance of developing insulin resistance. In

turn, this increases the odds of becoming overweight, obese and diabetic. (When people switch to a low-carbohydrate diet for all the health benefits mentioned elsewhere in this book, their insulin levels drop and their excretion of salt increases. A low-carbohydrate, real-food diet that avoids processed food will be low in salt and incur increased salt loss. It is essential, therefore, to add salt to our food. The slightly unwell feeling that people sometimes experience when switching to low-carbohydrate is usually caused by salt loss and rectified by more salt.)

Our bodies know when salt levels are too low. Receptors in the brain recognise the deficit and trigger a craving for salt but, according to DiNicolantonio, because we are conditioned to avoid salt we sometimes mistake this signal as a craving for sugar. Sometimes we eat more sugar when we should be eating more salt.

When we are trying to maintain normal blood-salt levels, in the absence of adequate dietary intake, we pull salt out of storage in the skin and bones. Calcium and magnesium are extracted from the bones, along with the sodium, then excreted in the urine. This weakens our bones and increases the likelihood of osteoporosis.

Iodine is an essential trace mineral that is necessary for our thyroid gland to function properly. Table salt usually has iodine added to it and naturally-occurring sea salt and rock salt contain a variety of trace minerals including iodine. So, if we limit our intake of salt, thus restricting our intake of iodine, this reduces the production of thyroid hormones. This leads to tiredness, fatigue, slowed metabolism and fat storage.

Low levels of salt are supposed to reduce blood pressure but they do something else: they increase heart rate. What advantage will anyone gain by a slight lowering of blood pressure when there is a measurable increase in heart beats per minute? Conversely, a higher intake of salt slows the heart rate which is of great benefit to anyone with heart problems.

Aldosterone is a hormone produced by the adrenal glands when salt levels get too low. It increases sodium retention but it does so at the expense of magnesium. We excrete more magnesium when aldosterone is raised. A deficit in sodium leads to a deficit in magnesium. Magnesium is an essential component of our energy production and this is one of the reasons a low-salt diet causes tiredness. Magnesium is also important in the mechanism of heartbeats. Calcium triggers heart muscle contraction and magnesium triggers the relaxation that follows. Atrial fibrillation is an uncomfortable and potentially dangerous condition where the top chambers of the heart beat very quickly. It is an increasing problem for older people but in some cases it can be remedied with an increase in magnesium. For some people, atrial fibrillation might be avoided with an adequate salt intake.

Salt restriction is bad for athletes. A good intake of salt increases blood volume and aids in the relaxation of blood vessels. Dilated blood vessels not only bring more oxygen, nutrients and energy to the muscles but also improve heat loss from the skin. The greatest heat loss during exercise comes from the evaporation of sweat and sweat contains salt. Plentiful salt allows for plentiful sweating which increases the loss of excess heat.

Who should we listen to?

The message that salt is bad for us has been repeated so often and for so long that it is firmly fixed in our minds and in the minds of doctors, journalists, nutritionists and the authorities. Public Health England condemned DiNicolantonio's book, *The Salt Fix,* when it was released in the UK. They said it was not only wrong but potentially dangerous. They claimed it would cost lives and good, reliable evidence showed that salt reduction reduced blood pressure. It is worth remembering that these are the same experts who recommend eating an impossible-to-measure 400 calories for breakfast and 600 calories for lunch and dinner, despite evidence from 60 years ago that this does not work. I have to say that I do not trust Public Health England to improve my health.

Someone I do trust is Dr Malcom Kendrick. On his website, he wrote a blog entitled *Salt is good for you* and this is the first paragraph:

"One of the most pervasive and stupid things that we are currently told to do is to reduce salt intake. This advice has never been based on controlled clinical studies, ever. Yet, as with the cholesterol myth, the dogma that we should all reduce salt intake has become impervious to facts. I find that the 'salt hypothesis' is rather like a monster from a 1950s B movie. Every time you attack it with evidence it simply shrugs it off and grows even stronger."

He is right; some people are convinced salt is bad for us because they are convinced salt is bad for us. Among so much conflicting advice who can we rely on? We can rely on ourselves, by which I mean our body's exceptional ability to look after itself. Receptors in the body monitor salt and blood volume levels. When they fall too low, the brain creates a sense of craving for salt, which we should not ignore. Salty foods will taste good when we need them but when we have high levels of salt already, the taste receptors on the tongue will become more sensitive to it and salty foods will taste too salty, which will encourage us to stop eating them. Millions of years of evolution have created the intricate and wonderful system of homeostasis that has kept us healthy without the input of 'experts'. We just need to trust it.

If you have any of the symptoms of salt deficiency such as loss of appetite; headache; nausea; vomiting; lack of energy and enthusiasm; muscle cramps and weakness; confusion; lack of muscle co-ordination; and even personality change, try taking more salt and see if it helps. Experiment and see what happens: it won't hurt you.

The biggest problem with food intake in Britain, and many other parts of the world, is the over-consumption of processed foods. If we want to be healthy, we have to stop eating over-processed, food-like substances and return to eating real food that comes from a farm, not a factory. Processed food invariably has a large amount of salt in it and it is this intake that the health authorities are worried about. Instead of worrying about the salt, they should be worried about the entire process of fake-food manufacture. People will often satisfy their salt craving by eating large quantities of crisps, tortillas and other processed snacks. These products have almost no nutritional value; they increase insulin levels; and often contain additives that we should not be eating.

Sea salt or rock salt are better options than table salt because they contain a wide range of essential minerals, which table salt does not. The best way to obtain adequate salt intake is to add it to real food, either during the cooking process or just before it is eaten. If you don't like green, leafy vegetables, or you cannot get your children to eat them because they taste bitter, sprinkle them with salt. The bitterness will disappear. To make them really appetising and nutritious, you should melt a knob of butter onto them along with the salt. Try it and see how much they both improve the flavour. Do this for your children and they may even to start to like kale, cabbage and brussels sprouts.

Summary:
- Salt has become vilified for no good reason. It is lumped together with sugar and fat as the cause of all our ailments. We would die without salt and fat, whereas we thrive without sugar.
- Our blood is a solution of salt and, if we are dehydrated, doctors drip a salt solution directly into our veins.
- Salt has been used as a food preservative for thousands of years.
- Processed food can contain a lot of salt but, if we care about our health, we should avoid processed food. When eating a low-carbohydrate, real-food diet we need to add salt to it and our taste buds should be the judge of how much is too much.

Chapter 8

A DIETARY GUIDE OF MISINFORMATION

The NHS website has a section called the *Eatwell Guide*, which has been written to help us understand what to eat for good health. Millions of people, meanwhile, are suffering from epidemics of obesity, diabetes, heart disease, cancer, auto-immune diseases, mental health problems and nutrient deficiencies. As a result of my research, I believe the *Eatwell Guide* contributes to all these problems, rather than solving them. I have already explained how the advice to eat a high-carbohydrate, low-fat diet has caused obesity and diabetes, but there are other fallacies in the guide we all need to be aware of. Before we get into those, I think it is important to understand the composition of our bodies.

What are we made of?
The food we eat has three benefits: it provides energy for all our activities; it provides the materials for growth and repair; and it provides the vitamins and minerals that allow our systems to function properly. We need to eat the things we are made of so we can grow into adults; rebuild all the cells that become damaged and die during the normal process of living; and replace all the minerals lost in sweat and urine each day. Our bodies are made of skin and bone, muscle and blood, and heart and lungs but, at the most basic level, we are just a collection of molecules. We are an exquisitely organised and interconnected collection of molecules but molecules nonetheless. A medicine we might take, to tackle a disease for example, is a specific molecule that will react with other molecules in our body to create a particular effect. Food is also made up from a variety of molecules and each of them has a distinct action within us.

Our food consists of three major groups: protein, fat and carbohydrate. These are known as macronutrients. We also need to eat a wide range of micronutrients made up of vitamins and

86

minerals. The macronutrients not only provide our energy and the structure of our bodies but are also involved in a wide range of systems, hormones and enzymes designed to keep our bodies running smoothly. We need the correct levels of all of them to function at our very best.

The word 'essential' has a specific meaning in the world of nutrition. Our liver can manufacture some of the molecules we need and, therefore, we do not have to eat them. These are referred to as non-essential foods. Other nutrients, which we cannot make, must be included in our diet and these are called essential because it is essential that we eat them. This can be slightly confusing because both groups may be essential to our health but only the ones we have to consume are called 'essential nutrients'. I have read articles where even qualified nutritionists sometimes get this wrong.

Protein

- Proteins can be made from any combination of twenty different amino acids: nine of these are essential amino acids and the other eleven can be made by the liver. We can create thousands of unique proteins by altering the combinations of all the different amino acids. All our muscles, connective tissues, skin, hair and organs are made of protein. Some of our hormones and enzymes are made of protein. The reading of our genetic code is controlled by proteins. Antibodies in our immune system are made from protein. Haemoglobin is a protein that transports oxygen in our blood and fats are transported by lipoproteins. Our skeletal muscle is the same substance as red meat. An average adult male is 42% red meat and an adult woman is typically 36% red meat. Some people have suggested that eating red meat can be harmful to our health, but surely it is illogical to think we can be harmed by something when more than a third of our bodies is made of it?

Fat

- Dietary fat consists of different molecules called fatty acids. They are referred to as lipids in scientific literature. There are three types: saturated, monounsaturated and polyunsaturated. Every natural source of dietary fat contains all three types. Fat plays a far greater role in our bodies than just the storage of excess energy. Seventy per cent of the structure of our brain is made from fat molecules. The membrane, or outer wall, of every cell in our body is made from fat. A third of all our cell membranes consist of cholesterol, which is a type of lipid. The membrane controls what goes in and out of each cell. The protective sheath around all our nerve fibres is made from fat. Vitamin D and all our sex hormones are made from fat molecules. Fat, or lipids, are used for energy but they are also essential for the integrity of our brains, nerves and cells. The idea that it is healthy to eat a low-fat diet, and starve our brains of the material it is made of, is unwise, to put it mildly. The recent huge increase in dementia and Alzheimer's disease may well turn out to be a direct result of the official advice to avoid dietary fat.

Carbohydrate
- Carbohydrate consists of various sugars. The most common sugar is glucose but our diets can also include fructose and galactose. Sucrose (table sugar) and lactose (from milk) are combinations of these, while starch (potato, bread, pasta, rice) is a long chain of attached glucose molecules. The only sugar our bodies use is glucose and its only purpose is to supply energy. There is no such thing as an essential carbohydrate because the liver can make glucose from both protein and fat. Nothing in the body is made from carbohydrate, unless you include the glycogen store, where excess glucose is kept. As there are no essential carbohydrates and no bodily structures are made of it, there is absolutely no need to eat carbohydrate. As long as we eat enough protein and fat, we can live a long and healthy life without ever consuming a single carbohydrate.

How can it possibly make sense for the dietary guidelines to recommend that all our meals consist of 65% carbohydrate when we don't need to eat any?

Vitamins

- Vitamins are classified as either water-soluble or fat-soluble. There are 13 vitamins that humans need: 4 fat-soluble (A, D, E, and K); and 9 water-soluble (8 B vitamins and vitamin C). The water-soluble vitamins are easily absorbed but the fat-soluble ones need fat in the diet to transport them into the body from the intestines. Vitamins have a wide range of essential functions ensuring the complex systems operating throughout our bodies run smoothly. A lack of certain vitamins can lead to dangerous deficiency diseases. It is essential that we eat fresh, unprocessed foods to ensure an adequate intake of vitamins.

Minerals

- Dietary minerals are chemical elements that are essential for the optimum function of our bodily systems. In order of abundance in the human body, they include: calcium, phosphorus, potassium, sodium, chlorine and magnesium. Others, known as trace elements because they are needed in small amounts, include: iron, cobalt, copper, zinc, manganese, molybdenum, iodine and selenium. As with vitamins, we need to eat unprocessed foods to obtain the minerals we need.

According to the *Eatwell Guide*, we are supposed to base all our meals on starchy foods such as bread and pasta. Both of these are made from grains of wheat and wheat is a type of grass. Other types of grass we eat include rye, barley, oats and maize. We are encouraged to choose wholegrains and boxes of breakfast cereal proclaim they are 'full of wholegrain goodness'. I think they use the term 'wholegrain' because it sounds similar to wholesome and the definition of wholesome is conducive to good health. Are wholegrain grass seeds conducive to good health? It turns out we are not birds nor insects and we did not evolve to eat grass seed. Our ancestors did not eat them until the development of agriculture about 10,000 years ago, which is like yesterday in terms of evolution.

History is always my starting point for nutritional research. The Ancient Egyptians were one of the first people to adopt large-scale crop growing and thanks to their papyrus manuscripts, statues, stone carvings and mummified bodies, we are able to learn a lot about their diet and their health. Records clearly show they ate a diet that a modern nutritionist would regard as excellent. You might even think the *Eatwell Guide* took its inspiration from ancient Egyptians. Their diet was based on a lot of bread and included fruits, vegetables and honey. They ate olives, sesame and flaxseeds. They added fish and waterfowl to this and very occasionally some red meat. There was no sugar and no refined or ultra-processed convenience food.

Autopsies and electronic scans have been performed on hundreds of mummies and they show very consistent results. The bread-eating Egyptians were fat and many of the males had Gynaecomastia, which is commonly referred to as 'man boobs'. They had terrible dental problems including abscesses, caries, missing teeth and ridges on the enamel, which indicates nutritional stress. Thickening of the arteries and calcification of the arteries was common, even among people who died as young as thirty. Some skulls show areas of small, pitted holes which indicates iron deficiency. They were smaller in stature than hunter-gatherer people from the same time period.

A document written in 1,550 BC, known as the *Ebers Papyrus*, contains the following sentence: "If you examine a man for illness in his cardia and he has pains in his arms and in one side of his cardia... it is death threatening him". Over three thousand years ago, they knew the symptoms of a heart attack and that must be because it was a common occurrence. And yet, these people were eating precisely the diet the NHS tells us to eat to avoid a heart attack. The problem, then and now, is a diet high in carbohydrate and low in animal fat and protein.

What is wrong with eating grass seed?

Every living thing tries to protect itself from harm and needs to reproduce. Animals can defend themselves in a variety of ways: fighting, fleeing, stinging, biting or curling into a ball like a hedgehog. Plants are just as keen on survival and reproduction but, because they cannot move, they use other tactics. Grains, beans, nuts and seeds are all 'baby' plants. Some plants surround their offspring with fruit because they want animals to eat them, transport them somewhere else and excrete them, unharmed, in fresh fertiliser. Grains, however, evolved to be dispersed by the wind and they do not want to be eaten by anything. They contain a variety of compounds that are designed to stop animals, including humans, from eating them.

- Lectins. Lectins are part of the plant's immune system and are activated when the plant is attacked. They are concentrated in the seeds, especially the bran. Lectins have been shown to damage human intestinal cells increasing the chance of 'leaky gut syndrome', which is associated with autoimmune diseases like rheumatoid arthritis, Celiac disease, type I diabetes, and multiple sclerosis.
  Lectins can cross into the bloodstream and bind to our own immune cells, which is another way they can increase allergies and autoimmune diseases.
- Gluten. Gluten is the collective name for a variety of proteins found in the seeds of wheat, rye and barley. These proteins contain sequences of amino acids we find very difficult to digest and, in susceptible people, gluten does great damage to the intestines causing Celiac disease.
- Gliadin. This is another protein that has been shown to disrupt the permeability of the gut wall, allowing things into the blood stream that should not be there. It is associated with, a surprisingly high, 79 autoimmune diseases. Some of the most troublesome include: ankylosing spondylitis; Celiac disease; Crohn's disease; fibromyalgia; juvenile arthritis; multiple sclerosis; psoriasis; and rheumatoid arthritis.

- Phytate. Phytates are produced by wheat and other grains to protect them from pests like fungi and insects. Such is their effectiveness, the agricultural industry has produced strains of wheat containing high levels of phytate, thus reducing the need for pesticides. The problem with phytates in your bread and cereal is that they bind strongly to mineral elements like iron, zinc, calcium and magnesium, which prevent these essential nutrients from being absorbed.

According to Dr. William Davis, who specialises in improving his patients' health through the removal of all wheat products from their diet, there are other reasons to avoid processed grass seed. In his book, *Wheat Belly*, he says that partially digested gliadin fragments act on the brain to increase appetite, causing weight gain; trigger behavioural outbursts in children with ADHD; increase the incidence of paranoia in schizophrenics; and cause anger and anxiety. Two slices of wholemeal bread will raise blood glucose levels higher than the same number of calories of sugar, thanks to a component called amylopectin A. Grains also contain hormone disrupters, which is why men's breasts enlarge and their testosterone levels drop, and why women with polycystic ovary syndrome improve without grains. Grains can also disrupt the normal balance of gut bacteria leading to irritable bowel syndrome.

The *Eatwell Guide* tells us not to skip breakfast. It says, "A healthy breakfast is an important part of a balanced diet, and provides some of the vitamins and minerals we need for good health. A wholegrain, lower-sugar cereal with fruit sliced over the top is a tasty and nutritious breakfast." It is interesting that they recommend 'lower-sugar' cereal and then suggest slicing fruit onto it. Fruit has a healthy reputation way beyond reality. Fruits have been developed to be sweeter and sweeter over recent years, and they are now extremely high in sugar. So, we are told to choose a lower-sugar cereal and then put high-sugar fruit on it. As I explain in the next chapter, breakfast cereals were invented precisely because they were low in nutrient value. We now know wheat-based cereals cause weight gain, mood swings, hormone disruption and an array of autoimmune diseases. What exactly do they mean by 'wholegrain goodness'? Why does the NHS recommend this when they could recommend eggs for breakfast? Eggs are cheap, versatile and quick to prepare; they are a fantastic source of protein, essential fats, vitamins and minerals, which are all easily absorbed. They are one of the most nutritious foods you can ever eat. Reading between the lines of NHS dietary advice, eggs are not recommended because they contain saturated fat and saturated fat can increase cholesterol levels. This, we have been incorrectly told, will increase the risk of heart disease and death.

In Chapter 4, I explained what causes heart disease and it is neither cholesterol nor saturated fat. NHS advice is so badly out of date it is embarrassing. A mother's breast milk has nearly the same percentage of saturated fat as eggs: between 2 and 2.5%. If you believe that saturated fat causes heart disease, you also have to believe that millions of years of evolution put saturated fat into breast milk because it wants babies to die of heart disease. How likely do you think that is?

What is fat?
There is a lot of confusion and misinformation about dietary fat, especially saturated fat, which has been demonised for no good reason. It is worth knowing the difference between saturated and unsaturated fats. All fats contain the same three elements: carbon, hydrogen and oxygen. As we can see in the following diagram, the carbon atoms (C) form a bond with their adjacent carbon atoms to create a row. Carbon always makes four connections to other atoms so they also make a bond with two hydrogen atoms (H), one on each side. The combination of oxygen (O), hydrogen and carbon at the end of these molecules is called a carboxyl group. This structure is very slightly acidic which is why these molecules are referred to as fatty acids.

A saturated fat is so called because it is saturated with hydrogen atoms: there is nowhere for more hydrogen atoms to connect. A monounsaturated fat has one position on the chain of carbon atoms where a double bond has been made between two carbon atoms. This can only happen when these two carbons are each lacking a hydrogen atom; therefore, the molecule is not saturated with hydrogen atoms. A polyunsaturated fat has two or more double bonds in the chain of carbon atoms.

Saturated Fatty Acid

Unsaturated Fatty Acid

As we can see in the diagram, the double bonds in unsaturated fatty acids cause the molecule to bend. Although they are represented here as two-dimensional drawings, in reality, they are three-dimensional structures. When a lot of the same molecules are present, the bend prevents them from stacking closely together. The saturated fats, on the other hand, are straight and these molecules can easily line up close to each other. Therefore, foods with a high percentage of saturated fat are more dense and will be solid at room temperature, whereas foods with a lot of poly-unsaturated fats are less dense because of the bends in the structure caused by double bonds. They are referred to as oils because they are liquid at room temperature. We never eat pure saturated fat nor pure unsaturated fat. Every source of dietary fat is a combination of saturated, monounsaturated and polyunsaturated fat. There are no exceptions to this rule, although the proportions of each type can vary greatly. Butter, for example, has more saturated fat than olive oil causing butter to be solid and olive oil to be liquid at room temperature. However, they both contain all three types of fat.

Every cell in our body has a membrane around it and this membrane is made of fat molecules stacked together. Do you remember the story of the three little pigs? Even they know it is much safer to have a solid wall around you than a flimsy one. A cell membrane made of at least 50% saturated fatty acids is more akin to a house made of bricks because the saturated fat molecules can sit close together; however, a membrane made of polyunsaturated fats is more akin to a house of straw, because their structure leaves gaps. If we eat too much polyunsaturated fat and too little saturated fat, we risk the integrity of all our cell membranes.[1]

The *Eatwell Guide* consistently tells us to avoid saturated fat because the authors still believe the disproven and discredited hypothesis about saturated fat, cholesterol and heart disease. There is now a considerable body of evidence showing this idea is wrong but the Guide refuses to accept it. If we go on the NHS website and type 'saturated fat' into their search box, we get a list of articles. If we open the top one entitled 'saturated fat', we get another list which includes coverage of scientific papers disputing the link to heart disease. There is one, published in 2013, entitled, *'Saturated fat link with heart disease questioned'* and refers to an article in the *British Medical Journal* by Dr. Aseem Malhotra, a London cardiologist. Dr Malhotra points out that many recent studies have shown no link with heart disease and some have shown saturated fat to be protective. He says that fear of cholesterol has caused millions of people to take statin drugs they do not need when sugar is the real culprit. The conclusion drawn by the NHS authors at the end of the article reads:

There is no need to change current advice. As with many things in life, the adage of "everything in moderation" applies to your fat consumption. The body needs small amounts of fat to help it work normally. But most of us eat too much saturated fat – about 20% more than the recommended maximum amount.
Current guidelines state that:

- *The average man should eat no more than 30g of saturated fat a day.*
- *The average woman should eat no more than 20g of saturated fat a day.*

In 2014 another article appeared on the NHS site, *'Saturated fats and heart disease link 'unproven'.* Researchers from Cambridge, Oxford and Bristol Universities pooled the results of 72 studies that had looked at the link between fatty acids and coronary disease. They found no significant evidence that saturated fats increase the risk of heart disease and no significant evidence that polyunsaturated fats protect the heart. At the end of this article the NHS says, "Current dietary guidelines remain unchanged. Even if saturated fats don't directly harm your heart, eating too much can lead to obesity, which in turn can damage it."

I can forgive anybody for making a mistake because we all make them. What I cannot forgive is the refusal to change your mind when it is proven that you are mistaken. The NHS response to the evidence of 72 studies, showing they are wrong, is like a bad parent who answers a child's question with, "because I say so". They have been aware of this evidence for years but continue to push their discredited dogma. I am astonished by their final sentence: it is so petty. They are admitting the new evidence about heart disease could be correct but insisting they are not wrong about saturated fat by suggesting too much makes us obese. There is no evidence saturated fat makes us fat. Obesity is caused by too much insulin, which is the result of too much sugar. Fat has no effect on insulin levels.

On the front page of the *Eatwell Guide*, there is a subheading, "Eat less saturated fat and sugar". They put these two things together as if they are equally bad for our health. They list nutritious foods like cheese, cream and butter as things to minimise because of their saturated fat content. Also on the list is the cooking fat lard, which they suggest should be replaced by polyunsaturated vegetable oils.

You can't get oil out of a vegetable
People always used to cook with natural fats found in lard, beef dripping, butter, ghee and, more recently, coconut oil. The incorrect demonisation of saturated fat has persuaded many to swap these traditional foods for liquids referred to as vegetable

oils. Everybody thinks vegetables are healthy, so it follows that vegetable oils will be healthy too. The trouble is vegetable oils don't come from vegetables: the name is a marketing con trick. They are created by extracting oil from plant seeds using an intensive industrial process by means of extreme heat, pressure or chemical solvents. We are told they are better for our health than traditional fats because they are high in polyunsaturated fats and low in saturated fat. No human being ever ate these substances until 1911, when the process of extraction was invented. Millions of years of evolution made us into exactly what we are. How can it possibly be true that a food entirely absent from our evolution is better for us than the foods we ate to become what we are today? The answer, of course, is they are not and their overconsumption has dire consequences for our health.

Vegetable oils should be referred to as *Industrial Seed Oils* because that is what they are. Common examples are corn oil, soybean oil, sunflower oil, safflower oil and rapeseed oil. They all contain a high percentage of polyunsaturated fat. As I explained above, these molecules contain multiple double bonds between carbon atoms. A double bond may sound as if it is stronger than a single bond but these are not physical structures, they are chemical attractions. A double bond is much less stable than a single bond because it is easy for an oxygen atom to break the bond and attach itself to the unsaturated carbon atoms in the molecule. This process is called oxidation. You can do an experiment at home if you are so inclined: put a tub of margarine, with the lid off, on a kitchen bench next to a block of unwrapped butter and leave them there for a week. The butter will be fine but the margarine will be rancid because the high content of polyunsaturated fats will have been oxidised by oxygen in the air. When we eat seed oils these reactive fatty acids are incorporated into our cell membranes and when our cell membranes are oxidised, the cells are damaged or die.

Omega 3 and omega 6 are both essential, polyunsaturated fatty acids. We need both of them, in equal proportions, to be healthy, and throughout history our food contained them in similar amounts. This is important because omega 3 has an anti-

97

inflammatory effect and omega 6 increase inflammation. Seed oils contain a very high concentration of inflammation-boosting omega 6 and they are so ubiquitous in modern food that we are consuming 16 times as much omega 6 as omega 3. This means we have much more systemic inflammation in our bodies than we used to. Inflammation is implicated in a long list of modern diseases, including the ever-increasing scourge of heart disease, diabetes, cancer, Alzheimer's disease, inflammatory bowel disease, fatty liver disease and rheumatoid arthritis.

However, this is not the only problem. Seed oils are often sold as 'cooking oil' and when they are heated to the high temperatures used in frying, they are oxidised to form toxic compounds called aldehydes. These are very reactive and damage proteins, hormones and enzymes. They also attack our DNA causing mutations that lead to cancer. A professor of chemical pathology at DeMontfort University, Martin Grootveld, said, "If a meal is fried in vegetable oil, it contains 100 to 200 times more toxic aldehydes than the normal daily limit allowed by the World Health Organization". When the same oil is used repeatedly, the aldehydes continue to increase. Before the advent of the *Eatwell Guide*, your local fish and chip shop would have fried in lard or dripping but now they are required, by Food Standards, to use seed oil and they cannot possibly afford to change it every day. Every time they heat the oil it becomes more toxic, and the same thing is going on in pubs and restaurants that serve any type of fried food. Some of these aldehydes stay in the oil and attach to the cooked food but some are volatile and escape into the air. People working in fast-food outlets and chip shops are breathing in these compounds all the time. Over recent years there has been a marked increase in lung cancer among women in Asia. They are not inhaling toxic chemicals from cigarettes because they rarely smoke; however, they are breathing in toxic aldehydes because, every day, they fry food in a wok using seed oils.

There is enough information to fill a book on why we should all avoid seed oils and the following is a small sample:

- Seed oils are included in virtually every item of processed food on the supermarket shelf. Even bread, which used to be made from just flour, water, salt and yeast, now contains seed oil.

- Formula milks for babies contain seed oils, usually as their second most prevalent ingredient.
- A six year trial of 850 elderly men, in a care home in Los Angeles in the 1960s, was designed to test if seed oils improved heart disease. The intervention group replaced animal fats with soy, corn, safflower and cottonseed oils. After 6 years the intervention group had lowered their cholesterol levels by 13%. However, twice as many men in that group had died of cancer, compared to the people eating animal fat.
- Linoleic acid is the main omega 6 in seed oils. It causes pre-fat cells to turn into mature fat cells, promoting the accumulation of body fat and leading to obesity. It also oxidises the surface of low-density lipoproteins (LDL), which increase the risk of damage to the endothelium of arteries, thus heightening the chance of heart disease and stroke.[2]
- A study published in *Clinical Nutrition* showed that the omega 6 in vegetable oils was associated with a sharp decrease in male fertility.[3]
- Age-related macular degeneration is the leading cause of blindness in the elderly and it is increasing. Research has shown that the ratio between omega 6 and omega 3 fats in the retina has a significant impact. The more omega 6 there is, compared to omega 3, the greater the risk of going blind. The only foods that create a significant imbalance are seed oils.
- There is a product called *Wate-On* which was heavily advertised in magazines from the 1930s to the 1960s. It was aimed at thin women and used headlines like, 'Men wouldn't look at me when I was skinny'; 'How to add glamorous curves to your figure'; and 'Gain weight – stop being skinny and tired'. The makers gave a money-back guarantee that *Wate-On* would easily add 4 or 5 pounds to your weight within a week. It clearly did what it claimed

because the adverts ran for decades. What did it contain? It was simply a mixture of glucose and maize oil, which is carbohydrate and vegetable oil.

I find it bewildering that the *Eatwell Guide* recommends that, along with copious amounts of carbohydrate, we eat and cook with seed oils. They call them vegetable oils but they are the industrial products that increase your chance of inflammation, cancer, obesity and blindness. However, they will probably reduce your total level of cholesterol but, as we have already learnt, cholesterol does not cause heart disease and elderly people have better health with higher levels of cholesterol. The *Eatwell Guide*, in my firm belief, is not a guide to eating well.

Summary:
- Our bodies consist of proteins and fats. Our skeletons are made of minerals and we need vitamins and minerals to function correctly. Nothing in our body is made of carbohydrate. The liver can make all the glucose we need for energy. Despite all this, the *Eatwell Guide* says we should ensure 60% of our food is carbohydrate. The over-consumption of carbohydrate is mainly responsible for the obesity epidemic.
- The 'Guide' is based on the incorrect theory that saturated fat causes heart disease. This fallacy leads to the recommendation to replace natural fat with the oil extracted from seeds. Seed oils are something we should all avoid because they promote weight gain and increase the risk of cancer.
- A diet based on cereals, pasta and bread contains a plethora of anti-nutrients, which increase the chance of intestinal problems and reduce the absorption of essential mineral

Chapter 9

RELIGION, CORRUPTION AND CENSORSHIP

Have you ever wondered where breakfast cereal came from? Nearly everybody eats it nowadays and we are told it is a wholesome way to start the day, but who invented it and why? It will probably come as no surprise to learn that the first breakfast cereal was invented by a man called John Harvey Kellogg in 1878. It will probably come as quite a surprise to learn why he did it.

Kellogg was an American medical doctor of some renown and you may be thinking that, as a doctor, he devised 'Corn Flakes' for sound nutritional reasons. Sadly, you could not be further from the truth. As well as being a doctor, he was also a religious zealot in the church of the Seventh Day Adventists. They take Christian scripture literally and have a strong emphasis on diet and health. Dr. Kellogg took these beliefs to extremes. Like many other members of his church, he regarded passion and sexual arousal as sins and the greatest sin of all was masturbation. He went to great lengths to try to stop it. He wrote a booklet entitled, *'The Rehabilitation of Masturbators'*, where he described the extreme measures, even mutilation, he used on both sexes to curtail this 'sin'. He was an advocate of circumcising young boys and applying phenol to a young woman's clitoris to make the dreaded habit much more difficult. He sometimes sewed silver thread into the foreskin of boys so that erections were painful. He had a wife but never consummated his marriage because he thought it was sinful, and they adopted their children.

'Corn Flakes' were invented as part of his strategy against self-gratification. The Seventh Day Adventists strongly believed that completely bland foods would decrease, or prevent, sexual arousal and that strong (nutrient-dense) foods, like meat, would increase physical excitement. So, 'Corn Flakes' were designed from the start to be as bland as possible in the belief that a lack of taste and nutritional quality would diminish normal human passions. His brother, William, who was less of a zealot and more of a business man, started the Kellogg's company to sell bland, processed flakes of corn. William wanted to add sugar to the flakes to make them palatable but John wanted blandness above anything else. Eventually, William got his way and they now come sprayed with sugar. To make them slightly more nutritious than the cardboard box they come in, they are also sprayed with a few vitamins. This allows the Kellogg's Company to make the dubious claim that their dried flakes of corn might be healthy.

I find it sad that millions of families all over the world give their children Kellogg's cereals every morning without realizing the sinister intentions behind their invention. The real irony is, that in a much less dramatic and obvious way, he is still managing to damage children's health and well-being with a daily dose of sugar-laden junk food.

The Seventh Day Adventists are vegetarians or vegans and heavily promote their beliefs about not eating meat. Veganism in America has its roots in the Seventh Day Adventist church. Their religious beliefs, which link passion, meat and sin together, seem to be impervious to both science and logic. However, they are good at business. Kellogg's has become a major global brand and in Australia and New Zealand, a company called Sanitarium dominate the market for breakfast cereals and vegetarian products. The 'Sanitarium Health and Well-being Company' is entirely owned by the Seventh Day Adventist church and because they are a church, they are not required to pay taxes on their profits. A fortunate position to be in considering they had an income of 204 million dollars in 2014. Have you heard the expression, 'breakfast is the most important meal of the day'? It sounds like a scientific fact but it is not. It is a marketing slogan designed to promote breakfast cereals and was invented by Miss Lenna Cooper, who was a protégé of John Kellogg.

A big selling point for breakfast cereals is their convenience: just tip them out of the box, into a bowl, pour milk on and eat. Are they good for us? No, they are highly processed and refined, with very little nutritional value and consisting almost entirely of carbohydrate. A bowl of Corn Flakes, for example, is 84% carbohydrate and all carbohydrates digest down into sugar molecules. As we have already discussed, a sudden intake of sugar leads to excessive insulin production, mood swings, fat storage and weight gain.

Corruption

Religious, puritanical zealotry about 'sin' gave us breakfast cereals over 100 years ago but that influence is still strong among nutritional advice. Lenna Cooper was very prominent and in 1917 she co-founded the American Dietetic Association (ADA), which was renamed the Academy of Nutrition and Dietetics (AND) in 2012. This organisation has guided nutritional advice for over 100 years in America and is often copied around the world. They claim to be devoted to "improving the nation's health" which they do by promoting a series of Nutrition Fact Sheets. The trouble is these fact sheets are 'sponsored' by companies from the processed food industry to the tune of 20,000 US dollars a time. Having paid for them, the companies take part in writing these documents. The Association then promotes them through its journal and on its website. In 2008 the ADA announced that the Coca-Cola Company had become an "ADA Partner" through its corporate-relations sponsorship programme. The ADA said that it "provides partners with a national platform, via ADA events and programs, with prominent access to key influencers, thought leaders and decision makers in the nutrition marketplace." The ADA's press release also pointed out that "the Coca-Cola Company will share their research findings with ADA members in forums such as professional meetings and scientific publications."

The American Dietetic Association and the British Dietetic Association insist that all dieticians are registered with them. It is no wonder that nutritional advice is so confusing and biased. How can we trust the organisations responsible for giving advice when they began with puritanical religion and morphed into tax-avoiding corporations which take large donations from the processed food industry?

Big corporations in the food and drinks industry go to great lengths to influence their customers and defend their products. Their actions go well beyond the sponsorship of Dietetic Associations. For instance, Coca-Cola funds a group of researchers known as the Global Energy Balance Network.[1] The scientists involved are paid millions of dollars by Coca-Cola to produce academic papers and news stories promoting the idea that weight loss is all about energy balance. We have already seen, in Chapter 3, that the 'calories in, calories out' theory of weight control was proven to be false back in 1956. Despite that evidence, since 2008 Coca-Cola has paid two of the founding members of the Global Energy Balance Network almost 4 million American dollars for various projects, according to reports printed in the New York Times. The message they are trying to promote is simple: 'it doesn't matter how much sugar you consume as long as you do enough exercise to burn it off'. This is a blatant lie that boosts the profits of a world-wide corporation and causes huge damage to the health of millions of people. Sadly, Coca-Cola are not the only ones doing this.

In 2016 an article was published in the *Journal of the American Medical Association*, by a group of researchers who had uncovered some previously unseen correspondence.[2] In the 1960s there was increasing evidence that sugar was a major contributor to heart disease. This was bad news for the sugar industry, so they did something about it. An organisation called the Sugar Research Foundation secretly paid two eminent Harvard University scientists to produce evidence that fat was the cause of heart disease and not sugar. One of these scientists was Dr. Frederick Stare who was chair of Harvard University's Public Health Nutrition Department. When someone as prestigious as Dr. Stare put his name to the idea that fat causes heart disease, everybody listened. The other paid scientist was Dr. Mark Hegsted, who was a professor in the same department. He ended up being even more influential than Dr. Stare because he was directly involved in writing the 1977 American Dietary Guidelines. It is a shameful story of both corporate and individual, financial greed which put money ahead of the truth. These people demonised healthy fat and sanctified unhealthy sugar and this fallacy eventually made millions of people obese. Although this happened a long time ago, it has only recently come to light. However, corporate influence is still everywhere.

The British Nutrition Foundation is registered as a charity and it provides a comprehensive array of nutritional advice. I think that its name, and its status as a charity, make the British Nutrition Foundation sound like an organisation we can all trust. The trouble is I no longer trust anybody in this business, so I looked into who the sponsors might be. In 2015 the Foundation was sponsored by, among others, Kellogg's, Tate and Lyle, Coca-Cola, Pepsi, British Sugar, McDonald's, Mars, KP Snacks and McCain. Can we expect the British Nutrition Foundation to give unbiased advice when their financial existence depends on maintaining the sponsorship of the world's biggest peddlers of sugar and ultra-processed, food-like substances?

Misinformation

One of the most deceitful and unethical practices in modern medicine is the use of relative risk instead of absolute risk. It is deliberately used to mislead us and we need to be able to recognise it when we see it. When the newspapers announce that taking 'snake oil' will reduce your chance of dying from exposure to 'cosmic radiation' by 50%, it sounds fantastic. Let's say that out of every one hundred people, two die this way each year but only one in every hundred die when they take 'snake oil'. To you and me, the difference between 2 out of 100 and 1 out of 100 is 1. We can see that the reduction of our absolute risk is 1%, which is fairly insignificant. However, the marketing department of the 'snake oil' company isn't interested in absolute risk. It looks at relative risk, which says that changing the death rate from 2 all the way down to 1 is a 50% reduction and it makes that claim in its advertising.

The marketing of the cholesterol lowering drug, Lipitor, is a real-life example of this statistical deception. The advertisements for Lipitor in medical journals and product brochures claim that the active ingredient, Atorvastatin, reduces death from heart attack by 36%.[3] This claim persuaded doctors all over the world to prescribe this statin to millions of people and Lipitor became the most financially successful drug in the history of the pharmaceutical industry, with sales in the region of 100 billion dollars.

The evidence for this claim came from a large, randomised, controlled study called the Anglo-Scandinavian Cardiac Outcomes Trial, in which people were split into two groups and given either Atorvastatin or a placebo. At the end of the trial Lipitor was claimed to be a life saver but if we look closely at the published results, we get a different picture. How many people did not have a heart attack or stroke? Among those taking the statin, 98.1% of all the thousands in the study had no heart-related problems. This looks good for the statins until we see that in the group taking the placebo, 97% had no cardiac events. In reality, the drug on trial was saving one person in every hundred from heart disease. Considering all the debilitating side effects of statins mentioned in Chapter 6, it is clear that a 1% reduction in risk simply isn't worth it. How did they come up with the much more interesting figure of 36%? The people taking a placebo died at a rate of 3% and the difference between them and the people on Lipitor was 1.1%. So, for no good reason that I can fathom, they have divided 1.1 by 3 and got a 36% relative risk reduction. To advertise the benefits of a drug using this method of calculation is, in my opinion, not just misleading but unethical and unscrupulous. And it goes on all the time.

There has been a recent and significant rise in the number of reports suggesting animal foods are dangerous for our health and an equivalent rise in the number of people eating less meat. This topic is covered in the next chapter but it requires a mention under the heading of 'misinformation'. Powerful vested interests have the opportunity to make fortunes by persuading everyone to eat plant-based foods. The genetically modified seeds for many crops, and the pesticides and herbicides that are sprayed on them, are both owned by a tiny number of corporations. Just as companies like Coca-Cola provide funding to promote the erroneous calories-in, calories-out theory, the agro-chemical business is very capable of misleading us over the benefits of plants compared to meat.

One of the tactics used by 'Big Business' is to suggest that the results of observational studies prove that meat increases the risk of certain diseases. I explained in Chapter 2 that an observational study cannot prove that one thing causes another and, as I will show, the evidence against meat comes from very weak, observational methods. The people who write about diet in newspapers appear, sometimes, to be unable to understand that an association is not a cause. It has become common to read the mantra that animal foods are bad for us, as if it were an undisputed fact. This is misinformation which I will rectify in the next chapter.

Censorship

In Chapter 2, I mentioned that the astronomer, Galileo Galilei, was found guilty of heresy by the Inquisition in 1633 and sentenced to imprisonment. This was later commuted to house arrest and that is where he spent the rest of his life. His 'crime' was to publish the truth about how the solar system operates. The authorities of the time were all religious men and they were not interested in his truth because they wanted to maintain their 'truth'. They found him guilty of heresy, which is a crime invented by the church to punish people who disagree with their doctrine.

In the 19th century a Hungarian doctor and obstetrician named Ignaz Semmelweis was concerned about the number of newborn babies dying from Puerperal Fever. After a period of meticulous record keeping, he discovered that the number of deaths could be drastically cut by the use of hand disinfection in hospital maternity wards. Puerperal fever (also known as Childbed fever) was common in mid-19th century hospitals and often fatal. While working in Vienna General Hospital's first Obstetrical Clinic, Semmelweis proposed, in 1847, the practice of washing hands with chlorinated lime solutions. He had noticed that doctors' wards had three times the mortality rate compared to midwives' wards. Doctors at the time would regularly go from an autopsy of a decaying body, to the birth of a child, without washing their hands.

Despite the publication of various reports, where hand washing reduced mortality to below 1%, Semmelweis's observations conflicted with the established scientific and medical opinions of the time. His ideas were rejected by the medical community, partly because Semmelweis couldn't explain why his method worked. Some doctors were offended by the suggestion that they should wash their hands and mocked him for it. Many of them believed that the hands of a doctor were also the hands of a gentleman and couldn't possibly be responsible for infant mortality. Such was the extent of his rejection that, in 1865, Semmelweis suffered a nervous breakdown and was committed to an asylum, where he died at the age of 47, after being beaten by the guards. Semmelweis's idea eventually earned widespread acceptance years after his death, when Louis Pasteur produced his germ theory and Joseph Lister, acting on the French microbiologist's research, practised and operated using hygienic methods. Lister was also rejected by the medical authorities in the early days of his career until his undeniable success became impossible to ignore.

People who are seen by themselves, and the wider community, as authorities in their field are often more interested in maintaining their position and status than accepting and adopting new ideas. Galileo, Semmelweis and Lister were all correct in their new ideas and all of them were censored by the establishment. Surely we now live in a more enlightened time and this sort of thing cannot still be happening? Sadly, it is most definitely happening now. Dietetic Associations around the world are the official authorities on nutrition and beware anyone who challenges their doctrine.

Gary Fettke is an Australian orthopaedic surgeon working in Tasmania. Most of his daily work consists of amputating the gangrenous feet of type 2 diabetics. This is work he does not enjoy. After doing his own research into the effect of diet on diabetes, he began advising his patients to avoid sugar and refined carbohydrates and to replace them with healthy fats from natural sources. Fettke wanted to prevent his patients from reaching the level of diabetic damage that required amputation. However, when a member of the Dietetic Association of Australia heard about this, he was reported to the Australian Health Practitioners Regulatory Authority (AHPRA). In 2016 he was banned from giving nutritional advice to any of his patients by AHPRA, which is the organisation in control of his registration to practice as a doctor.[4] In their message to him they said: "There is nothing associated with your medical training or education that makes you an expert or authority in the field of nutrition, diabetes or cancer. Even if, in the future, your views on the benefits of the Low Carbohydrate, High Fat (LCHF) lifestyle become the accepted best medical practice this does not change the fundamental fact that you are not suitably trained or educated as a medical practitioner to be providing advice or recommendations on this topic."

Apparently, he is sufficiently well trained to cut off people's feet but is not trained to prevent them from needing a life-changing amputation. This is so typical of the 'Authorities'. If you possess a certificate, given to you by the 'Authorities', that states you are an expert in your field, then you are an expert. If you do not have their certificate, you are not an expert and you are not entitled to give people any advice. The fact that your advice may be saving lives and limbs is irrelevant. What always matters most to the people in charge is the maintenance of their status. They are more concerned with saving face than saving lives. I am pleased to be able to report that in 2018, after a great deal of negative publicity for the AHPRA, the ban on Fettke giving nutritional advice to his patients was lifted.

For many years Professor Tim Noakes has been at the forefront of the LCHF movement in South Africa, where it is referred to as Banting, after William Banting. In 2014 a mother asked him on Twitter how she could adapt the diet he recommended for her baby because she was worried about excessive wind if the baby had too much dairy and cauliflower. He replied: "Baby doesn't eat the dairy and cauliflower, just very healthy high fat breast milk. Key is to ween baby onto LCHF". This tweet put him into a legal battle lasting four years. A complaint against Noakes was made to the Health Profession's Council of South Africa (HPCSA), his regulatory body, by dietician Claire Strydom, who was then chairwoman of the Association of Dieticians of SA.

The charge against him was whether or not Noakes had been giving "unconventional advice" over social media and whether he had been treating the mother's baby as a patient, without conducting an examination. Doctors cannot treat patients over social media. The entire process from complaint to verdict lasted three years; expert witnesses were flown in from around the world and individuals gave evidence that lasted for days. In 2017 Noakes was found not guilty of any of the charges but the saga was still not over because the HPCSA appealed against the verdict and the process began again. The appeal found there was no doctor-patient relationship between Noakes and the mother, who had used Twitter to ask for general advice, and in 2018 Noakes also won the appeal.

During the hearing, Noakes's lawyers produced e-mails they had discovered through the South African equivalent of Freedom of Information rules. The e-mails were between the dietitian, Strydom, and a professor of dietetics at North-West University in which they discussed a plan to complain about Noakes before the tweet in question was even posted. Noakes's legal team argued that the two had planned to take him down and waited until they had found a tweet to use against him. This pre-planned complaint against someone, who is clearly helping people in South Africa to lose weight and become healthy, caused this highly respected Professor to suffer years of anguish, have his reputation tarnished and would have cost him millions had his two advocates, Mike van der Nest and Rocky Ramdass, not acted for him without charging a fee.

Another process that can bring about a type of censorship is the Peer Review. When a scientist wants their work published in a scientific journal, it is subjected to a review by other scientists working in the same field. This scrutiny by one's peers may seem, at first, like a good idea because they would be able to recognise mistakes using their own experience. Also, when the work has been reviewed by other experts, it has more credibility. This may work well most of the time; however, what will happen when somebody comes up with an entirely new solution to a problem that demonstrates that all the other people in that field are wrong? How likely is it that a group of specialists is going to allow the publication of material that will destroy their own life's work? Galileo, Semmelweiss and Yudkin had their careers destroyed by the opinion of their peers, despite the fact that they were correct and their peers were wrong.

Who can we trust?

Unfortunately, it appears that we can trust very little of the information we are given. I hope you will trust me and believe that I am telling you the truth, as much as I know it. You will have to decide for yourselves if I am trustworthy from the arguments and information I provide. I want you to be sceptical about so much information that I realise you may be sceptical about the things I say. I want you to think about all the information in this book and decide for yourself what may or may not be true, just as I have done for the last few years.

If you are thinking that I am too sceptical, I will finish this chapter with the words of Marcia Angell, who resigned after twenty years as the editor of one of America's leading scientific journals.[5] "It is simply no longer possible to believe much of the clinical research that is published, or to rely on the judgement of trusted physicians or authoritative medical guidelines. I take no pleasure in this conclusion, which I reached slowly and reluctantly over my two decades as an editor of the New England Journal of Medicine."

Summary:
- Religious beliefs about 'sin' created vegetarianism. Zealotry about 'sin' created breakfast cereals.
- The Seventh Day Adventist Church still exerts a great influence on nutritional advice around the world.

- Global corporations in the food and drink industry fund scientists to deflect blame away from their sugar-laden, highly processed products and onto natural foods that we have eaten for millennia.
- Brave individuals who challenge the status quo are denigrated, censored, suspended or taken to court.

Chapter 10

VEGANISM AND HEALTH

Vegetarians are people who do not eat meat or fish. Their diet consists mainly of plant foods but they will often consume animal products like milk, cheese, yoghurt and eggs. Some of them are pescatarians and they will include fish in their diet. Vegans take things a step further and exclude all animal foods. They only consume plant foods and some will also refuse to use any animal products such as wearing leather shoes or belts. There has been a surge of interest in veganism in recent times. Reports in the media suggest that a vegan, or plant-based, diet is more healthy than an omnivore diet; it is kinder to animals and it is better for the environment. Are these claims true? In this chapter, I write about the health aspects of plant-based diets and, in the next chapter, I will examine their impact on the environment.

In Chapter 1, I asked the question, 'why are so many people ill?' I have spent several years looking at a huge range of research with an open mind. Because of my background as an Olympic Marathon runner, I began with a bias towards the idea that people need to take more exercise for better health. After studying the evidence, it has become clear to me that, while exercise is extremely important, the food we eat is the crucial factor in our health. As a pharmacist, I was taught, and believed, that cholesterol and salt have to be reduced to avoid heart disease. Thanks to an open and inquisitive approach, I have found evidence about these two essential nutrients, which has changed my belief completely and I now know that what I was taught was wrong. It is important for us all to know if the claims made by vegans are actually true, so I have studied the evidence with the same open and scientific mind that I have tried to use throughout this book. I have always eaten a fairly typical, mixed, omnivore diet but after investigating the evidence for a vegan diet, I have made changes to the way I eat. I now consume considerably more meat, eggs and cheese and fewer plant foods than I did before.

If somebody wants to be a vegan they are entitled to make that decision for themselves and I respect freedom of choice. I believe that people should be able to do whatever they want, but with one very important caveat: what they do should not prevent anyone else from doing what they want. People are free to choose veganism if they want to but they are not entitled to tell everyone else that it is healthier than a diet which includes food from animals. All the evidence I describe in this chapter makes it very clear to me that veganism is not an appropriate diet for our species.

Newspapers, and other media, appear to be giving vegetarianism and veganism a disproportionate level of coverage. A survey in America, by the Humane Research Council in 2014, stated that only 2% of the population avoids meat and of those only 0.5% are vegan. Headlines that proclaim a 'huge surge in people turning vegan' actually mean a few people have given up meat. The Humane Research Council's report also stated that five in every six vegetarians give up their abstinence and eventually return to eating meat.[1] If you are planning to become vegan and you are not dissuaded by my writing, before you do so, please read a book called, *The Vegetarian Myth* by Lierre Keith. She was vegetarian for 20 years. She returned to eating meat after she realised that her diet had permanently damaged her health.

I do not want to tell you what to believe. I want to give you the information so you can decide for yourself. The British philosopher, Bertrand Russell, once said, "The whole problem with the world is that fools and fanatics are always so certain of themselves, and wiser people so full of doubts." I do not expect to persuade any vegans to change their mind with this chapter; however, I do hope to inform all the people who are beginning to believe there may be some truth in the frequent reports about the harmful effects of meat. Surveys have shown that more and more people are reducing the amount of meat they eat. As I will explain, these stories are driven by vested interests who are using that old ploy of 'tell people something often enough and they will start to believe it'.

What does history tell us?

In Chapter 3, I explained how we evolved to be the dominant species on the planet by chasing after, and eating, large animals. The nutrient-dense, easily-digestible meat, fat and organs of animals gave us the energy and sustenance to grow large brains and, in accordance with Kleiber's Law, smaller intestines. Our tremendous ability to run long distances and lose excessive body heat through sweat on our hairless skin can only be explained by the need to chase food. Cave paintings from 50,000 years ago show men in pursuit of large animals. There are no cave paintings dedicated to the glory of plant food. Indigenous populations still survive in a wide range of remote places and none of these are vegan; some are entirely carnivorous, like the traditional Inuit of northern Canada and the Masai of Kenya; while some others are more omnivorous. Studies have shown that three quarters of all hunter-gatherer groups worldwide get 60% of their energy from animal foods. If any indigenous people ever tried to live on a plant-only diet, they either gave up or died out. All the evidence suggests that we evolved to be the way we are because of a diet dominated by nutrient-dense animal food.

As I mentioned in the previous chapter, the avoidance of meat began in America around 1860 with the Seventh Day Adventist Church and their illogical belief that sexual arousal was a sin. They believed that meat was especially arousing and bland food decreased sexual desire. In their opinion, the promotion of vegetarianism was the most effective way of denying as many people as possible the pleasure and bonding experienced in an intimate, physical relationship. Their advocacy of plant-based diets had nothing to do with a person's health and everything to do with their idea of 'sin'.

In Britain, veganism began with a man called Donald Watson who founded the Vegan Society in 1944. He is credited with coining the word 'vegan' which he created by joining the beginning and end of the word *vegetarian*. He was an animal rights campaigner whose interest in veganism began when he witnessed the slaughter of a pig on a farm. He campaigned for a meat-free diet because he thought farming was cruel to animals, not because he thought it was more healthy. It appears that the story about veganism being healthy is a later addition to the creed, which has coincided with an attack on the health benefits of animal foods.

Is meat good or bad?
Humans have been eating meat for hundreds of thousands of years and, clearly, we have not died out. The recent surge in doubt about meat has been fuelled by a World Health Organisation (WHO) report in 2015, which declared, *"the consumption of red meat is probably carcinogenic to humans."* This, of course, was the headline but if we look at the details, we see that it is only for, *"colorectal cancer and based on limited evidence."* Where does the evidence come from? The International Agency for Research on Cancer, IARC, considered a selection of observational studies on meat consumption and disease. We already know that observational studies cannot prove that one thing causes another but this was the evidence they used.[2] The declared level of risk for meat causing colorectal cancer was between 1.17 and 1.18. The chance of anybody developing colorectal cancer in their lifetime is 4.5%. If the IARC information is reliable (which I will show it is not), the regular consumption of red meat increases your risk to 5.3%. We live in an increasingly carcinogenic world where the air we breathe, the water we drink, the processed food we eat and the household cleaners we use, contain a host of chemicals which all increase the risk of cancer. How can it make sense to avoid the most nutrient-dense food we have for a possible 0.8% reduction in the risk of getting a fairly rare cancer?

I have previously mentioned the Grade system for ranking the strength of evidence in observational studies. Two distinguished professors, who were involved in the development of Grade, have published an article entitled, *Mistaken advice on red meat and cancer.* Gordon Guyatt and Benjamin Djulbegovic insist that relative risk needs to be 5 or higher to give researchers any confidence to declare that a particular food is causing a particular disease. A risk of 1.18 cannot be used as proof of causation. In their article they said:

"The WHO has done the public a disservice in abandoning Grade in its evaluation of the evidence, and greatly overstating confidence in a causal connection between red meat and cancer. Recent decades are littered with policies based on weak relative risks which, when properly tested in clinical trials, had to be reversed.... Bias against red meat is another factor, easily perceivable in the scientific literature and the popular press..... Randomised clinical trials provide far more trustworthy evidence. It is perplexing that the WHO document does not mention two large, multi-year trials; the Polyp Prevention Trial and the Women's Health Initiative. In both trials the intervention group significantly decreased red meat and processed meat but researchers found no effect on any type of cancer."

Dr Georgia Ede is an American psychologist who specialises in the effects of nutrition on brain function. In Britain, Dr Zoe Harcombe has a PhD in nutrition. Dr Frank Mitloehner is an Animal Science specialist in California. Independently, all three of them have examined the research used by IARC and they each state these studies are unable to demonstrate that meat is a probable cause of colorectal cancer. In other words, the World Health Organisation has published a report which states that eating the food our species has been eating for hundreds of thousands of years is a cause of death and they have based it on research which does not prove that conclusion at all.

What is going on? We are being lied to: that is what is going on. We were lied to about saturated fat, about high-carbohydrate diets, about cholesterol, about vegetable oils, about calories and about salt. When we understand how many lies we have been told, it becomes much easier to realise that this is just another enormous lie. To get to the bottom of what is going on, we always need to ask questions.

Why did IARC investigate a link between meat and cancer in the first place? Had there been a sudden increase in deaths from eating meat? The IARC website says that an 'International Advisory Panel' suggested they should investigate this topic. We already know who controls and funds dietary and nutritional organisations: it is Big Business. Global corporations use these organisations to further their ambitions because the only thing they care about is *their wealth*, not *your health*. Whoever the 'International Advisory Panel' actually are, we can be confident they are not an independent group of free-thinking medical practitioners.

Once the idea that meat may be bad for our health has been repeated often enough to filter into people's minds, the real attack begins. In late 2018 a report was published in a scientific journal by Dr Marco Springmann of Oxford University.[3] He argued that a tax on meat was needed to reduce consumption. He claimed this would save thousands of lives every year and save the planet from climate change. This was very widely reported in all the media. What I noticed from all the coverage was none of the journalists challenged any of the data he was using nor searched for any conflicts of interest. I have already explained that the WHO announcement is scientific codswallop, so why is an Oxford University researcher making these claims? Dr Springmann is a dedicated vegan and has been for over ten years. This does not mean that he cannot be correct but it does mean that he has a self-declared bias and we should, therefore, be sceptical. If his work is biased and the research he uses is not reliable, how did he get it published? His paper was published in a journal called PloS One. A little investigation reveals that PloS One was founded by a man called Dr Pat Brown, who is also a fervent vegan. He is a man on a mission to turn the entire world vegan. In a 2009 interview with Jane Gitschier he said: "I am serious, and I'm going to do my sabbatical on this: I am going to devote myself, for a year, to trying to the maximum extent possible to eliminate animal farming on the planet Earth." He also happens to be the CEO of the company that makes the 'Impossible Burger', which is an ultra-processed, vegan substitute for a beef burger. That looks like a conflict of interest to me.

This entire business of blaming meat for ill health and climate change is an agenda. It is not fact and it is not remotely sensible but it is an all-out campaign to fool gullible people and most of us are very gullible when a scientist, in a position of authority, tells us what he wants us to believe. Militant vegans have realised they cannot demonstrate that their diet is healthy, so they have decided to attack meat and all other animal foods. Unfortunately, the people who write about nutrition in newspapers are not scientists; they are journalists who either do not have the time, or do not know how, to check and verify the research papers they report on. These naive correspondents are a dream come true for the vested interests that are trying to deceive us. Most of them happily trot out all the false dogma of the last few decades and their latest mantra is, 'we all need to eat less meat'. We are at the stage where we cannot rely on newspapers for health or dietary advice. We have to discover the truth for ourselves.

Some of the media bias towards veganism can be explained by this example. In 2017 an American organisation called the Open Philanthropy Project gave $886,600 to the Guardian newspaper, via its U.S. fundraising arm, Guardian.org.[4] In return for the money, the Guardian runs weekly articles on the worst cases of poor practice and cruelty in animal agriculture. Why would they do that? The Open Philanthropy Project is an investor in the company that makes the plant-based Impossible Burger. It is much more cost effective for companies to buy editorials than to place advertisements. When people see an advertisement, they know they are being sold to but when they read an article they are more likely to believe it is a true picture.

Guardian.org was set up by the Scott Trust, which is the sole shareholder in the Guardian Media Group. According to the Guardian's UK website: "The Scott Trust forms part of a unique ownership structure for the Guardian that ensures editorial interests remain free of commercial pressures". How do they reconcile that statement with the fact that Guardian.org was set up to raise money from commercial interests in return for editorial?

Carnivores
Something that is rarely mentioned in this debate is the evidence from carnivore groups. The Inuit of northern Canada have traditionally lived happily and healthily with no plant foods in

their diet for most of the year. Their typical diet consists of fish, seal meat, whale meat and blubber. They were studied extensively in the early 20th century. In 1902 Dr Samuel Hutton began treating people at a missionary hospital on the northern coast of Labrador. He reported that he could not find any cancer, asthma, appendicitis nor other "modern" diseases among the Inuit who were isolated from European settlements.

Weston Price was a Canadian dentist who wondered if modern diets were causing all the crooked and decaying teeth he was witnessing every day. In the 1930s he visited the Inuit and found that, not only were their jaws wide enough to fit all their teeth without overlap, there was no tooth decay and they all appeared to be strong and healthy.

Dr Vilhjalmur Stefansson was an Arctic explorer who spent most of his time, between 1906 and 1916, living with the Inuit in their ice houses in the far north. Like them, he lived exclusively on local animal foods. When he returned to New York and told everyone about his diet and the excellent health of the Inuit, he was met with a lot of scepticism. To prove what he said was true, he and his co-explorer, Dr. Karsten Anderson, volunteered to live on nothing but meat for an entire year. They spent the first two weeks eating under laboratory conditions and, for the rest of the year, paid observers ensured they ate nothing but meat. They both remained in excellent health throughout the trial, except for one short period when the researchers persuaded Stefansson to eat only lean meat. He became unwell within a few days but returned to good health as soon as he returned to eating the large amounts of animal fat that he had requested at the beginning of the experiment. (As I have said before, 'lean meat' was a political compromise and it has never had science behind it. In fact, there is a condition called 'rabbit starvation' because some explorers, who were only able to find rabbits as food, died from malnutrition. Rabbit meat is extremely lean and does not contain enough fat to sustain life.[5])

These polar explorers are not the only people thriving on a meat-only diet. Many people are discovering that avoiding plant foods and eating only animal foods greatly improves their health in some circumstances. Mikhaila Peterson is a young woman who was diagnosed with the auto-immune disease, Juvenile Rheumatoid Arthritis, when she was seven. Over the following years she developed depression, extreme fatigue and severe acne. She was prescribed a lot of medication which did not solve her problems. In desperation, she tried the carnivore diet: she now eats only beef, salt and water. All of her health problems have gone.

Deficiencies in a Vegan diet

Vegan diets are devoid of vitamin B12. Without this essential vitamin our bodies cannot make red blood cells, the myelin sheath around our brain circuits, nor even DNA. Animal foods are the only reliable source of B12 and it is vital for vegans to take supplements of this vitamin, or eat yeast-based foods like Marmite, to avoid serious deficiencies. Research has shown that 68% of vegetarians and 83% of vegans are deficient in B12, compared to 5% of omnivores. How serious can this deficiency be?

A paper in the scientific journal, *Human and Experimental Toxicology*, reported the admission to hospital in 2012 of a 16 year old girl who had stopped eating; couldn't sleep or walk; had decreased self-care and high blood pressure; was having fits, hallucinations and a depressive mood. Her blood tests were normal except for very low vitamin B12. After receiving injections of B12, all of her problems disappeared within a week. In 2016 the *Journal of Babol University* reported the case of a middle-aged man who was suffering from restlessness, nightmares, visual and auditory hallucinations, delusional beliefs, suicidal ideas, insomnia and anorexia. He was also cured with vitamin B12 injections.

A vegan mother who is deficient in B12, and other vitamins, will create a baby with those deficiencies and will provide breast milk which lacks the necessary nutrition for proper child development. Frederick Leroy is a Belgian academic who specialises in food studies. He has compiled a list of hospital case reports on the problems suffered by babies breastfed by vegan mothers.[6] It is a long and tragic list but typical defects include: anaemia; failure to thrive; repetitive vomiting; dystonia (movement disorder); hypotony (dangerously low pressure in the eye); failure of psychomotor development; muscular atrophy; brain atrophy; irreversible neurological deterioration; tremor; and microcephaly (failure of the skull to develop to its full size). If vegan diets do this much damage to children, how can they possibly be the best diet for adults?

A couple in Sydney, Australia, were taken to court in early 2018 and charged with (a) failing to provide for a child; (b) causing serious injury; and (c) grievous bodily harm. Their child was suffering from rickets and was considerably below the average weight and height for his age. The parents had fed the boy a strict vegan diet. A year earlier a Belgian court had found parents guilty of causing the death of their seven-month-old son, Lucas, through neglect. His organs had shrunk to half their normal size and he died malnourished and dehydrated after being fed 'vegetable milk' made from oats, buckwheat, rice and quinoa. In 2016 a one year old boy in Milan was removed from the custody of his parents because the vegan diet they were feeding him left him severely malnourished. In Canada, a boy of 14 months died from malnutrition, along with a severe skin infection, gangrene, hypothermia and extremely low weight and height for his age. His parents were convicted, in 2018, of criminal negligence causing death. They are both members of the Seventh Day Adventist Church and killed their child with a totally unsuitable vegan diet.

I am extremely concerned that, for some people, veganism has become a quasi-religious doctrine and they feel compelled to follow their ideology, even when it causes clear and significant harm to their own children. I am not the only one who thinks a vegan diet is completely unsuitable for children. The Federal Commission for Nutrition in Switzerland stated in their 2018 report: *"The positive effects of a vegan diet on health cannot be proven, but there are relevant risks regarding nutritional deficiencies. Children and pregnant women are advised against adopting a vegan diet due to those risks."*

Across the border from Switzerland, the German Nutrition Society have stated: *"With a pure plant-based diet, it is difficult or impossible to attain an adequate supply of some nutrients. The most critical nutrient is vitamin B12. Other potentially critical nutrients in a vegan diet include essential amino acids, long-chain omega 3 fatty acids, vitamins B6 and D, and the minerals calcium, iron, iodine, zinc and selenium. The German Nutrition Society does not recommend a vegan diet for pregnant women, lactating women, infants, children or adolescents. Persons who nevertheless wish to follow a vegan diet should permanently take a vitamin B12 supplement, pay attention to an adequate intake of nutrients, especially critical nutrients, and possibly use fortified foods or dietary supplements."*

Nutrient availability

Vegans maintain that a carefully chosen, plant-based diet contains all the protein, vitamins (except for B12) and minerals required for health. This is another variation of thinking 'the sun goes round the earth' because it appears to be correct. In laboratory tests, plants can be shown to contain protein, vitamins and minerals. The problem, which is not easy to see, is a thing called bioavailability. Just because a plant contains certain nutrients does not mean that we can access them, absorb them and use them.

Plant foods are lower in dietary fat than animal foods and this leads to the poor absorption of fat soluble vitamins, A, D, E and K. Plants do not contain vitamin A in the form of retinol, which we use. They contain carotenoids which have to be converted to the active form. This process is considerably harder than obtaining retinol from animals. Our bodies use a form of vitamin D called D3, which we make from sunshine or obtain from animal foods. Plants contain D2, which has to be converted to the active form. Vitamin K is really two vitamins: K1 is needed for blood clot formation; but K2, which is essential for the function of brain cells, cell membranes and the deposition of calcium into our bones, is only available in its active form, known as MK-4, in animal foods. Vegans can supplement this with a bacterial form of K2 by eating fermented soy.

Iodine is an essential building block in the thyroid hormone, which is critical in brain development and maintenance, as well as for energy levels. Plant foods are low in iodine compared to most animal foods. Lack of iodine, particularly in early life, stunts body and brain growth. According to studies, iodine deficiency affects two billion people, and is the most common, preventable cause of intellectual disabilities in the world.

Iron is needed for oxygen transport but is also critical for brain function. Plants contain a form of iron that is much harder to absorb than the 'heme' iron found in meat. Zinc is another essential mineral that is hard to absorb from plants. A Swiss study showed that 47% of vegans are deficient in zinc compared to 10% of omnivores.[7]

It is harder for vegans to get the protein they need. As I explained in Chapter 8, there are 20 amino acids that we use to build proteins. We can make 11 of them but we have to eat the other nine. Animal foods, such as meat, poultry, fish, eggs and dairy, are considered to be complete sources of protein because they contain all of the essential amino acids we need to function effectively. Plant protein sources, such as beans, lentils and nuts are considered to be incomplete, as they lack one or more of these essential amino acids. Some people claim soy protein is complete. However, two essential amino acids are only found in small quantities in soy, which means it is not comparable to animal protein.

If you are thinking you can get over that problem by eating a lot of soy protein, you need to be aware that soy also contains molecules called phytoestrogens. As the name suggests, they are very similar molecules to the female hormone oestrogen and they can disrupt the normal function of our naturally occurring hormones.[8] The latest research on their effect in the human body is inconclusive. However, a lot of baby formula milk is now made with genetically modified soy protein and research in animals has shown some worrying results. In April 2010 researchers at Russia's *Institute of Ecology and Evolution* found that after feeding hamsters genetically modified soy, over three generations, most of the third generation of animals had lost the ability to have babies. They also suffered slower growth, a high mortality rate among the pups, and a high incidence of a rare phenomenon of hair growing inside their mouths.[9]

Brain food

Two thirds of our brains are made of fat molecules. Making up 20% of all that fat is an omega 3 fatty acid known as DHA, which is absolutely vital for brain function. According to Professor Crawford of Imperial College: "It maintains the integrity of the blood-brain barrier and mitochondrial membranes. It is essential for the transmission of signals across synapses and it acts as a semiconductor in the mitochondria. It turns sunlight striking the retina into the electric signal that the brain deciphers as sight." There is no DHA in plant food; it can only be obtained from animal foods. Another omega 3 fatty acid that is not available in plants is EPA. This has strong, anti-inflammatory properties and, as we know, many of our modern diseases are caused, or made worse, by too much inflammation.

Plants contain an omega 3 known as ALA, which has no function in the body. Some of it can be converted into EPA and DHA but it is a very inefficient process and leaves vegans well below optimum levels. Studies have shown that, compared to meat eaters, EPA levels are 28% lower in vegetarians and 53% lower in vegans. DHA levels are 31% lower in vegetarians and 59% lower in vegans, compared to meat eaters. Dr Simon Dyall, a lipid research scientist, has said, "DHA plays a unique and indispensable role in the neural signalling that is essential for higher intelligence." If our intelligence depends upon a compound only found in animal foods, it cannot be wise to eliminate it.

Research has shown that vegans and vegetarians tend to be more likely to suffer from depression, low mood and anxiety than meat eaters. A study published in *Ecology, Food and Nutrition* [10] stated: "The differences we found are consistent with other research that suggests that vegetarians are less psychologically well-adjusted than non-vegetarians." It is proven that vegans, and to a lesser extent vegetarians, have less than optimal levels of many essential nutrients. A paper published in *Current Psychiatry Reports* in 2013 encouraged mental health experts to consider nutrient deficiencies when treating their patients. The authors,

Ramsey and Muskin, produced a list of symptoms known to be caused by vitamin deficiencies:

- B1. Memory impairment, confusion, lack of coordination
- B2. Fatigue, cracked lips, sore throat
- B6. Convulsions, migraine, chronic pain, depression
- B9. Loss of appetite, weakness, palpitations, behavioural disorders
- B12 Depression, irritability, fatigue, anaemia, shortness of breath
- A. Decreased immunity, blindness
- D. Rickets, osteoporosis, muscle twitching
- E. Neuropathy, myopathy, weakness, retinal damage

In the United Kingdom, and many parts of the world, there is a growing mental health crisis, especially among young people. Our Government has promised to make extra funds available to provide counselling and therapy. What they should do is to speak out against the inadequacies of a plant-based diet and encourage everyone to eat real, unprocessed food with plenty of meat, fish, eggs and cheese. The trouble is this goes against their official dogma that still, despite all the evidence, promotes a high-carbohydrate, low-fat diet.

Summary:
- Our species evolved into what we are today because our ancestors ate lots of meat for hundreds of thousands of years.
- There are no indigenous tribes eating a vegan diet.
- The World Health Organisation's conclusion that meat causes cancer is refuted by independent researchers. The WHO ignored trials that disproved their findings.
- Groups eating an entirely carnivorous diet display excellent health.
- Vegan diets are deficient in essential nutrients like vitamins B12, A and D and omega 3 fatty acids EPA and DHA.

- Vegan propaganda is rampant in the media and is sometimes paid for by the processed-food industry.

Chapter 11

VEGANISM AND THE ENVIRONMENT

I strongly disagree with vegans who claim their diet is more healthy than an omnivore diet. However, I am in accord with their concerns over animal welfare. The worst cases of factory farming are awful; it is a system driven entirely by the desire to produce as much cheap food as possible. It shows scant regard for the welfare of the animals reared for food. If these creatures are going to feed us, we should show them respect and allow them to live a life that at least resembles their natural behaviour. The Bushmen of the Kalahari, who still hunt by chasing a prey until it collapses from heat exhaustion, perform a ceremony of respect over the animal's body as soon as it dies. They fully understand the reality of the circle of life on Earth and they accept that something has to die for others to live. This knowledge does not make them cruel; it makes them compassionate. Whilst I agree with vegan concerns about animal welfare, I wish they would campaign against the worst aspects of animal farming practices rather than put an end to all animal farming.

The worst examples of unnatural animal food production are known as concentrated animal feeding operations, or CAFOs. They are common in the United States where they produce cheap beef, pork and chicken. As the name implies, the animals are crowded together in cramped spaces. Cattle are kept in small pens with no grass beneath their feet. They are injected with antibiotics and fed a diet high in grains and corn that they have not evolved to eat. The excrement from these enormous feedlots is a serious problem. It does not go back into the ground as it should, but is stored in huge lagoons that can contaminate rivers and water supplies, causing a danger to public health. Corporate greed drives the appalling standards in CAFOs but the company executives claim they produce nutrient-dense food at a cheap price, which is what people want. Environmentalists point out that the system is rigged because the damage done to the environment, the waterways and human health is always paid for by the taxpayers, not by the companies creating the mess. When that is taken into account, the meat is not cheap at all.

CAFOs provide animal rights' enthusiasts and vegans with the opportunity to campaign against all animal farming. In 2018 it was reported that cattle CAFOs had begun to operate in Britain. I call upon the Secretary of State for Environment, Food and Rural Affairs to make these factory farms illegal in the UK. They are bad for the animals; they are bad for the environment; and because the animals are stressed, drugged and fed an unnatural diet, they provide poor quality food for people.

Proper animal welfare, which benefits the environment, is achievable if it is done correctly. In fact, as I will explain, it is essential. I have previously mentioned the huge importance of balance, or homeostasis, to our health and welfare. Not only does every creature have its own internal equilibrium but so does the entire biosphere. Life on Earth has evolved to exist in a state of self-correcting stability, which has worked beautifully for millions of years. Plants grow in fertile soil; herbivore animals eat the plants; and carnivore animals eat the herbivores. Our species can be counted among the carnivores. The meat in our diet comes mainly from ruminant animals like cattle, sheep and deer that exclusively eat plants. Other ruminants, which we don't usually see on the menu, include goats, bison, elk, giraffes and camels.

A ruminant is so called because it has a different digestive system to ours. Instead of one stomach, it has four compartments in its stomach, one of which is called the rumen. A cow, for example, eats grass and other plants that typically grow in a meadow. These plants consist mainly of a long chain carbohydrate called cellulose. We cannot live by eating grass because we do not possess the enzymes to digest cellulose. Interestingly, neither does the cow; however, its rumen is teeming with bacteria that convert cellulose into fatty acids and protein, which the cow absorbs. Ruminant animals are able to convert an abundant substance, grass, which is totally inedible to us, into meat and meat is the most nutrient dense food there is.

Vegan activists want to persuade everybody that this amazing conversion performed by ruminants is bad for the planet. Why do they think this? The bacteria in the rumen digest cellulose by a process called anaerobic fermentation and a by-product of this is methane, which the cows belch into the atmosphere. Methane is said to be a greenhouse gas and it is claimed that too much of it increases the possibility of global warming. They try to tell us that if we all stop eating meat and we get rid of millions of ruminants, we will reduce greenhouse gas emissions back down to a safe level. Instead of blaming the trillions of tons of fossil fuels burnt by the oil, gas and coal industries in the last hundred years, they want to blame cows and sheep instead. Ruminant animals have been on the Earth for 50 million years and they have burped methane throughout that vast length of time without 'destroying the planet'. They also play a vital role in the homeostasis of grasslands, which I will come to. What could go wrong, if we do what people like Springmann suggest, and remove one piece of an exquisitely balanced eco-system?

The notion that 'cows burp methane; methane is a greenhouse gas; and, therefore, we need to get rid of cows,' is an absolutely classic example of 'the sun goes round the earth' thinking. It seems so logical but it is completely wrong because of something we cannot see happening. The thing we cannot see is underground: it is the ecology of soil. Before I explain that, I want to do some arithmetic.

Grass grows by taking CO_2 out of the air. With the help of energy from sunshine and water from rainfall, grass converts atmospheric CO_2 into molecules of carbon, hydrogen and oxygen. Some of these carbohydrate molecules, called cellulose, are used to create new blades of grass and some, which are more simple sugars, are passed down the plant and into the roots. To keep the arithmetic simple let's assume a blade of grass absorbs 100 molecules of CO_2 and that 80 of them are used for growth and 20 of those carbon atoms go down to the roots, where they will stay if the ground is left undisturbed.

Constance the cow comes along and eats all of those 80 carbon atoms in the grass. The bacteria in her rumen get to work and convert plant cellulose into the fatty acids and proteins that Constance needs to grow. A by-product of this process is methane gas which is produced at a rate of approximately 5% of the food Constance eats. Therefore for every 100 molecules of CO2 absorbed by grass, cows return 4 or 5 of them to the air as methane. Simple arithmetic and basic biology show it is impossible for cows, or sheep, to add greenhouse gases to the atmosphere. They simply recycle a few of them.

It is possible to calculate the amount of methane in the atmosphere over the last 1,000 years by examining the concentration of methane held in ice cores. According to the website, methanelevels.org, the atmospheric methane level was 678 parts per billion in the year AD 1,100. With very little fluctuation in between, it was exactly the same in 1645 and 1725. During those 625 years, before the European settlers made too much difference to the American landscape, it is estimated that herds of 75 million bison, elk and deer were roaming, and belching, across the vast grasslands of the mid-west without making any difference to atmospheric methane.

Why did methane levels remain constant for hundreds of years with millions of burping ruminants? Methane is short lived. It only stays in the atmosphere for about ten years before it is converted to carbon dioxide. If the number of animals stays the same, then the level of methane they produce will always stay the same. Rainforests, wetlands and rice paddies also produce methane, when vegetation rots without access to oxygen. When has anybody ever told us to eat less rice to 'save the planet from climate change'? The atmospheric level of methane reached 1,000 in 1930 and rose exponentially to 1,482 in 1980 and reached 1,857 by 2017. For hundreds of years it stayed the same but in the last couple of centuries it has risen sharply. When I see these figures and then hear so-called experts saying we have to 'eat less meat' to reverse climate change, I know with absolute certainty that this is an agenda and I am being lied to.

Soil ecology

Have you ever wondered where fertile soil comes from? Just like everything in the biosphere, it evolved in harmony with living things. When the settlers and farmers from Europe arrived in the middle of America, they found the most fertile soil they had ever seen and to their amazement it was between six and ten feet deep. For thousands of years those 75 million bison and deer had roamed the land, eating the grass and other plants that grew there. But they did it in a very specific way. Just like antelopes in Africa keep together in a tight herd for protection from lions and tigers, bison and deer in North America travelled in herds to lessen the danger of attack from wolves and pumas.

When a large group of ruminants find new pasture they eat the top of the grass and urinate and defecate onto it. They don't want to eat their own dung, so they move on before they overgraze that area. The removal of the top part of a plant stimulates it to grow. (If they eat it all the way down to the roots it weakens the plant too much, which is why grazing is good and overgrazing is bad.) Their excretions fertilise the land and their hooves break up the surface, just enough to help rainfall soak into the ground. After they move on, the plants grow stronger and they absorb carbon dioxide from the air. They use this carbon to create their own structure and, importantly, to make simple sugar molecules which travel down the plant and into their roots.

We all have trillions of bacteria in our intestines and they perform a vital role in our health. In a similar way, there are trillions of bacteria and fungi in a handful of soil and they form an essential symbiotic relationship with the plants. The fungi are known as mycorrhizal fungi and they perform an extraordinary job.[1] They consist of a network of long, very fine strands called hyphae. These filaments colonise the root system of nearly all plants and feed on the sugar molecules which the plants create. In return, the fungi provide the plants with water and minerals. The structure of the fungi gives them a greater reach and surface area than the plants' roots can achieve by themselves. The hyphae also excrete enzymes that increase the absorption of minerals. Not only this, but the same network of filaments can colonise the roots of many plants simultaneously, allowing different plants to share nutrients. This underground network has been shown to make plants more resistant to disease. For example, when one plant in the network is attacked by aphids, all the others are stimulated to produce volatile organic compounds that attract the natural predators of the aphid.

The fungi also help to create clumps of soil called aggregates and these greatly improve the soil's ability to retain water. Bacteria in the soil colonise the fungal network and some of them are able to capture nitrogen and add that element to the mix. Healthy soil also contains bacteria called methanotrophs which capture and use methane for their growth. It is hard to measure how much methane they extract from the air but they are part of the extraordinary homeostasis thriving beneath our feet.

Fossil records have shown that mycorrhizal fungi and plants have been enjoying their mutually beneficial relationship for at least 400 million years. The carbon that plants take out of the air and pass down through their roots to the fungi and bacteria below ground is a constant process which helps to store carbon in the soil. This process makes new soil. It is the reason the settlers in America found fertile soil up to ten feet deep. Many people are aware that carbon can be stored in the atmosphere and levels are getting higher. We may also be aware that carbon dioxide dissolves in sea water and too much of it makes the oceans less alkaline. (It does not make them acidic.) Not so many people realise that soil is also an important carbon storage facility and herds of animals are necessary to maximise that process.

Where do ruminant animals fit into this ecosystem? A wild area of grassland has many different plant species growing on it. Some of them grow much taller than the others. If they are left to grow to their full height, they block out the sun from the shorter plants, which then wither and die. This creates a layer of dead plant matter on top of the soil known as thatch. Too much thatch holds water and prevents rain from seeping down into the ground. The roots of the surviving plants grow upwards in search of the water but away from the fungal network and nutrient rich soil. This weakens both the taller plants and the mycorrhizal fungi. This entire problem is avoided when ruminant animals come by and eat the tops off each plant, allowing sunlight to reach them all, fertilise the ground and move on. So what is the answer to the question I asked earlier about what could go wrong if we removed ruminants from the ecosystem? The grasslands, which co-evolved with plant-eating animals, would wither and die: slowly degrading into deserts.

Human interference

What is the quickest way to damage the incredible symbiosis that exists between animals, plants, bacteria and fungi? The answer is ploughing, or tilling as they call it in America. People used to believe that turning over the soil, and putting the organic matter from the plants underground, would increase the fertility of the soil. That was before we knew about mycorrhizal fungi. Ploughing rips apart the network of hyphae that is so important to soil fertility. It also exposes a great deal of the carbon, which is stored beneath ground, to the air and that carbon becomes oxidised to form carbon dioxide, a potent greenhouse gas. The effect of ploughing on global warming is something I have never seen in the calculations of greenhouse gas emissions from animal farming but if we are all going to eat a plant-based diet, as the vegan activists insist we should, farmers will do even more ploughing.

My daily walk takes me along the banks of one of England's rivers. When there has been little rain, the water is clean enough to see the stones on the river bed. After heavy rain, the water level rises considerably and it becomes distinctly brown and completely opaque. This brown material is soil that has been washed off ploughed fields by the rain. This is happening in every river around the world where fields are ploughed for crops. According to the United Nations Convention to Combat Desertification, a third of the planet's land is severely degraded and fertile soil is being lost at the rate of 24 billion tons a year. Soil isn't washed away from land that is covered by grass because the extensive root system holds it in place. Grassland absorbs rainfall, improving fertility and reducing both drought and floods.[2]

Fields used repeatedly for crop growing become less fertile and need to have man-made fertiliser added to the soil. The use of large amounts of nitrogen and phosphate-rich fertilisers has increased yields for many farmers and it has become an enormous business for agrochemical companies. The Food and Agriculture Organisation of the United Nations says the amount of fertiliser, used by farmers around the world, surpassed 200 million tons in 2018. This increase in yields for farmers would appear to be a good thing and, in the short run, it is. The problem is the long term use of fertilisers. Firstly, the application of too much nitrogen has been shown to reduce yields over time: it can cause excessive growth of the whole plant, rather than just the edible part; and it also disrupts the balance of other nutrients. In addition, excess nitrogen washes off the land, along with the topsoil, and into the rivers where it disrupts the natural balance. Waterways are normally kept free from too much nitrogen by denitrifying bacteria converting the nitrogen to gas, which then escapes into the atmosphere. Vast amounts of fertiliser, washing into streams, overwhelm these bacteria and the nitrogen level rises. This nutrient-rich water encourages algae to grow in enormous blooms, sucking all the oxygen out of the water and leaving 'dead zones' where no fish can survive. Around the world, the area of these dead zones has quadrupled since 1950.[3] At the mouth of the Mississippi River, in the Gulf of Mexico, there is a dead zone of up to 7,000 square miles.

Plants for food are typically grown in large mono-crop fields, which can be planted and harvested with enormous machines. Hedgerows are ripped out to make the fields bigger and more 'efficient'. Weeds and insect pests have to be eliminated so the crop is sprayed with pesticides and herbicides. The drastic decline we have witnessed in birds, bees and butterflies is the result of the loss of habitat and the application of toxic chemicals, caused by modern, crop-growing practices. In September 2019, the New York Times reported a loss of 3 billion birds in the USA and Canada during the previous 50 years. When people decide to become vegan because they do not want other living creatures to die for their food, they have an image in mind of a cow in a slaughterhouse. It would seem they are totally unaware of all the hundreds of field mice, hedgehogs, birds, bees, butterflies and fish killed to provide the vegetables on their plate.

What would happen to the planet if the activists get their way and we all become vegan? Millions of people will starve to death because excessive crop farming will turn vast tracts of land into desert. If you are thinking that wouldn't happen, I need to explain that it already has. A hundred years ago farmers on the American plains were growing wheat on as much land as they could because wheat prices were high. They did so much ploughing and planting of a single crop, they turned those deep, fertile soils I mentioned earlier, into what became known as the 'dust bowl'. The grass, which had covered those prairies for a million years, was turned over; the fungal network was destroyed; the land dried out; and when a period of drought came, the soil was turned to dust and blown by the wind, across the country, as huge, dark clouds. Thousands of farmers were made bankrupt and there was an enormous exodus of people from the mid-west to California, in search of work. The US Government bought millions of acres of land and replanted it with the original prairie grass.[4]

Some reports of the 'dust bowl' say the famers were unlucky because the weather brought a drought. Recent research, however, suggests their actions may have caused it. Rain forests are so called because they create their own rain. Plants release water vapour into the air, from their leaves, by a process called transpiration. Large areas of dense vegetation, like a rain forest, produce so much water-vapour that when it cools high in the atmosphere, it falls back as rain. Studies have shown that large areas of grass can do the same thing. When we swap the grass for a ploughed field, the process stops.

Our species is known as Homo Sapiens, which means 'wise human'. It appears we are not quite as wise as we would like to think we are. It seems the more we interfere with the natural world, the worse we make it. When it comes to the ecology of our planet which one of these are you inclined to trust: an academic, self-appointed armchair analyst or 400 million years of evolution?

The people I trust are the ones who accept reality and work in harmony with nature.

The real solution to our problems

Grassland, savannah, prairie, plains, steppe, pampas and shrubland are names from around the world to describe large areas of land covered mainly in grass, with perhaps a few trees and shrubs. They are not forests and they are not suitable for intensive agriculture. They occur all over the world and account for 45% of the earth's land surface. They are very important and many of them are in trouble because they are starting to degrade and turn slowly into deserts. The breakdown of grassland happens when small patches of grass die and the soil beneath is exposed to the air. When the sun shines on green grass, the energy is absorbed and used but when it falls on bare soil, it acts as heat. As the soil warms it loses moisture through evaporation, which makes it harder for any plants to grow there. These dry patches of soil draw moisture from surrounding areas, reducing the water available for the remaining plants. Rainfall on bare earth is not absorbed but runs off the ground instead. Slowly but surely, the patches of bare soil grow larger, which accelerates the degradation of the land. It is estimated that 23% of all grasslands are somewhat degraded.

The overgrazing of grasslands by ruminant animals has been shown to be another cause of desertification. It was decided that resting the land from any type of grazing would solve the problem but wherever this was tried, it made matters worse. Luckily for us all, people who understand the evolution of grasslands have demonstrated how to solve this problem. Allan Savory is a pioneer in grassland rehabilitation. He is an ecologist and farmer in Zimbabwe. Most of the land he farms was severely degraded until he applied what he calls, 'holistic management'. Instead of reducing the number of cows and sheep on his land, he increased it considerably. He moved the animals, in tight herds, to a new piece of land on a daily basis, which almost perfectly mimics the natural movement of all the wild herds that created and sustained the grasslands for millions of years. He has given a TED

Talk on his work, which has been watched by 3.5 million people. In the presentation, he shows before and after photographs of brown, almost-bare scrubland, which is then transformed into areas of vibrant plant growth. This is brought about entirely by the actions of ruminant animal behaviour of grazing, fertilising and moving on.

The remarkable ability of ruminant animals to transform poor quality land into healthy pasture has huge importance in the world today. Millions of people live in semi-desert areas and often suffer from malnutrition. If they can be taught to use Allan Savory's techniques, they can create better grazing. This will allow them to farm more animals, which will provide more income and higher quality food. The huge increase in plant life, created by holistic management, increases the sequestration of carbon from the air into storage in the ground and it does it without any need for artificial fertiliser.

Research projects in America have measured soil carbon levels before and after controlled grazing experiments. A small sample of this research is listed below:

1. A study was performed by the School of Ecology, at the University of Georgia, and published in *Nature Communications* in 2015. It involved three farms in the south east of America. After switching to management intensive grazing, they were able to sequester 3.2 tons of carbon per year per acre.[5]

2. At West Wind Farm, in West Virginia, they use carefully controlled, rotational grazing. Researchers used soil samples to demonstrate that the farm sequestered 15 tons of carbon dioxide per acre over a four year period.[6]

3. A study by the University of South Dakota was published under the title, *'Green House Gas Mitigation Potential of Different Grazing Strategies'*. Their analysis of various grazing systems found that converting to rotational, multi-paddock grazing sequestered 2 tons of carbon per year per acre.

Based on these measured and confirmed numbers, it is possible that holistically managed herds of ruminant animals could take 21,000 tons of carbon out of the air every year, and store it underground, if they are grazed on 12 billion acres of the world's grassland. In thirteen years the Earth's atmosphere would have returned to pre-industrial levels and we would have vastly more productive land.

Vegan activists and fanatics want to rid the world of cows and sheep for the sake of reducing greenhouse gas emissions. They are wrong about vegan diets being healthy. They are also wrong about the effects of ruminant animals on the environment when the animals are reared correctly on permanent grasslands, which is typically the case on British farms. Please do not be taken in by journalists who trot out the dogma of the day: 'we all need to eat less meat'. The truth is the exact opposite. We all need to eat plenty of animal meat and fats to be healthy and we need many more grazing animals, properly managed and living a healthy life, to maintain the ecology of our beautiful planet.

Summary:
- Vegan activists claim we should eat less meat to protect the environment but ruminant animals have been a vital part of the ecology of our planet for millions of years.
- Cows burp methane but this is part of a cyclical process that has no effect on the Earth's climate.
- Holistically managed ruminants are essential to the health of vast tracts of grassland. They fertilise the soil and help plants to sequester carbon underground.
- Ploughing fields for crops damages the fertility of the soil and releases carbon dioxide. It also allows top soil to be washed away by rainfall.
- Artificial fertilisers leech into streams and rivers causing dead zones where no fish can survive.

Chapter 12

EXERCISE IS VITAL

I read this message on a sign somewhere and have always remembered it: "Exercise is a celebration of what you can do; not a punishment for something you ate." In Chapter 4, I explained that exercise is a very poor way to lose weight because the calories used by jogging or walking typically come from the glycogen store and make no difference to your excess weight, which is stored as fat. It seems, however, that a lot of people still believe that the main reason to exercise is to lose weight. The truth is that you cannot outrun a bad diet but that does not mean you should not exercise. There are multiple benefits to regular physical exercise. We evolved to be the way we are because, for hundreds of thousands of years, our ancestors chased after the animals they ate. Exercise is vital for our physical and mental health.

Mental health

Many studies have been performed to examine the link between exercise and mood. These have shown that people who exercise regularly have fewer symptoms of depression and anxiety than those who don't exercise. Medium intensity exercise can be an effective treatment on its own for mild to moderate depression. Sixteen weeks of regular exercise was shown to be just as effective as anti-depressant medication in treating older people who were not exercising previously.[1] People with depression, who had partially responded to anti-depressants, were found to increase their improvement when exercise was added to the medication. The research has shown that both aerobic exercise (such as walking, cycling or running) and strength training (such as weight lifting) can help to treat depression. Fairly strenuous exercise triggers the production of endorphins. These are the body's natural pain killers and they reduce the discomfort of vigorous effort and can also elevate our mood.[2]

A lot of people associate exercise with going to the gym but research has shown that exercising outdoors in 'green spaces' greatly benefits the mood-elevating effects of physical activity.[3] We have spent 99.9% of the previous million years being physically active outside and researchers believe there is a strong genetic link, deep within us, which reacts positively when we are in contact with nature. Studies have shown that exercising in the great outdoors is not only much cheaper than the gym, but also much better for you. Whether you like running, cycling or walking, doing it outside in green spaces, rather than on urban concrete, boosts your mood, lowers your stress levels and makes you feel more revitalised and energetic. In fact, just five minutes of activity outside in the presence of nature can have an immediate (and lasting) effect on your mental health; and, if you are exercising near some water, this effect is even greater. (I can attest to this. During my running career I ran thousands of miles and always used woodland or riverside footpaths whenever I could. On dry, sunny days these runs made me feel wonderful. My regular walk now takes me through a wood and returns home on a riverside path and, while I cover the ground a lot more slowly, I still get a feeling of comfort and joy.)

Plenty of research has shown that young people are becoming increasingly disconnected from nature. They spend far less time outdoors in green spaces than previous generations and they are suffering from record levels of mental illness. The negative effects of too much screen time are part of the problem but so is the lack of 'green exercise'. In the next chapter, I discuss the mood-lifting benefits of the bright light we are exposed to when we exercise outside in daylight.

Memory

As discussed in the chapter on evolution, regular, prolonged exercise increases the production of Brain Derived Neurotrophic Factor (BDNF), which is essential for the creation of memories and the maintenance and integrity of brain structures. In Chapter 16, I describe how physically fit school children do better academically than unfit children because of their superior brain chemistry. This effect also helps people of every age to have better memories and better problem-solving abilities. Middle-aged people, at the height of their careers, do better if they are physically fit and this benefit can carry on into old age.[4] In a rare study of people in their nineties, researchers measured levels of dementia and mobility in the residents of a care home. Men and women who were unable to lift themselves out of a chair were 30 times more likely to have dementia than people of the same age who could comfortably get out of a chair and walk the length of the corridor.[5]

Exercise maintains muscle mass and muscle mass is essential for the process that triggers the increase in BDNF, which in turn maintains the brain and reduces the chance of dementia. Instead of participating in sedentary activities, with little mental stimulation, elderly people would benefit greatly by doing some weight training.

Physical fitness

We all know that regular exercise improves our fitness but what does that really mean? It means increased physical strength to lift heavier objects or to climb anything from stairs to mountains more easily. It builds endurance which allows us to be active for longer. It strengthens heart muscle and improves the efficiency of the whole cardiovascular system allowing us to do more strenuous activity before we get out of breath. Regular exercise can also reduce blood pressure, which decreases the chance of heart disease.

As we get older, we all tend to lose muscle via a process called sarcopenia. Extra muscle mass improves balance and smooth movement. This reduces the chance of falling over, which can lead to possible fractures and further immobility. Strong muscles and smooth movement also inhibit the development of arthritis in our joints. Improved insulin sensitivity, which reduces the chance of diabetes, dementia and some cancers, is another important benefit of muscle maintenance. Exercise increases muscle tone and definition, which makes us not only look and feel better but also boosts our self-esteem.

Sex life

Increased self-esteem and a toned body make us all feel more attractive, thus reducing any inhibitions we may have about being naked. According to Dr Tina Penhollow of Florida Atlantic University, "regular exercise increases sexual arousal, the frequency of intimate activities, the performance of those activities and the percentage of satisfying orgasms".

The strength and flexibility gained from frequent exercise improve sexual performance as does the increased blood flow that comes from a healthy cardiovascular system. Dr Penhollow also points out that regular exercise improves our mood and reduces stress, both of which have positive effects on our libido.

Osteoporosis

Osteoporosis is a condition that weakens bones, making them fragile and more likely to break. It develops slowly over several years and is often only diagnosed when a minor fall, or sudden impact, causes a bone fracture. The most common fractures happen in the wrist and hips. Three million people in the UK suffer from osteoporosis. Loss of bone density is a natural occurrence as we get older and is accelerated by smoking and too much alcohol.

In the same way that our muscles become stronger when subjected to the stress of exercise, our bones become stronger when they are put under pressure. The best way to avoid osteoporosis in old age is to have strong, dense bones when we are younger. Our bones respond to regular, weight-bearing exercise by increasing their density which, in turn, increases their strength. If we build strong bones in our youth and middle-age, we can afford to lose some bone density without developing fragile bones in old age.

Sleep

Regular exercise can also improve sleep quality.[6] It increases the time spent in deep sleep which is the most restorative sleep phase.

Deep sleep helps to boost the immune system and control stress and anxiety. In addition to improving the quality of sleep, exercise can also lead to an increased duration of your nightly rest. Being physically active helps you to feel more tired and ready to rest at the end of the day. A regular exercise routine can help to reduce stress levels. Stress is a common cause of sleep problems, including trouble falling asleep and sleeping restlessly during the night. As we have seen, exercise is a potent remedy for anxiety and other mood disorders; just 5 minutes of exercise can trigger an anti-anxiety response in the body. Research shows that mind-body exercises, such as yoga, pilates and stretching, can help to lower cortisol levels and reduce blood pressure, as well as having positive effects on mood. Feeling anxious makes it very difficult to fall asleep.

Evidence indicates that exercise can be an effective therapy for insomnia, without the need for medication. It reduces insomnia by decreasing arousal, anxiety and depressive symptoms. Studies have also found that exercise can help to lower the severity of sleep-disordered breathing and may also reduce the severity of obstructive sleep apnoea. Finally, exercise may have benefits for insomnia by its effects on circadian rhythms. The most profound effect on our body clocks comes from exercising earlier in the day. Exercise just before bedtime interferes with sleep in some people because it makes us too warm and mentally alert.

Types of exercise
In recent years there have a been a lot of positive recommendations for high intensity, interval training, or HIIT, as it is known. Proponents of this form of activity claim that we can become physically fit with just five minutes a day of intense exercise. The method involves short bursts of flat-out activity, with short rests in between each effort. It is often done on a static bike, rowing machine or treadmill in a gym but can be done running up a steep hill or even up and down your staircase. Flat-out efforts involve working our major muscle groups very hard and they respond by becoming stronger. It also makes our heart rate shoot up, thus stimulating and strengthening our cardiac muscle. The

considerable increase in oxygen requirements, during intense exercise, improves our ability to transport and utilise this vital element. Our muscles become stronger and our cardiovascular system becomes more efficient.

This is all good news but I need to add a word of caution. I think middle-aged and older people who are not fit and carry excess weight should be very careful doing such intensive activity. Pushing our heart as fast as it will go, vastly increases the pressure and turbulent flow of blood in the arteries and we know this can lead to the rupture of plaque, if we happen to have any.

Five minutes of exercise may sound perfect for people who always feel short of time but it is worth remembering that the benefits of HIIT are almost entirely found in measures of physical fitness. Such short bursts do not allow enough time for the development of meaningful levels of neurotrophic factors to be produced. To improve our memory, cognitive abilities and to ward off dementia, we are better off doing longer and, therefore, less strenuous exercise. At least fifteen minutes of continuous, aerobic exercise of medium intensity appears to be the minimum requirement for meaningful production of BDNF.

As any athletes who are reading this will know, the best approach is to combine both types of exercise into our routine. A period of time spent on longer but slower aerobic activity increases our endurance and fitness, whilst building the resilience to cope with more demanding exercise in the future. If we try to do high intensity work without a good base of all-round fitness, we are going to find it extremely difficult. But, if we are already in good shape, HIIT activity can take our fitness levels forward rapidly.

I mention this often but only because it is so important: we evolved into who we are because of all the running our ancestors did. Exercise, therefore, is not optional. We all need to exercise if we want to live a long and healthy life. The Government, for reasons known only to itself, invariably refers to exercise as sport. I am one of the millions of people who loves competitive sport but I am fully aware that many people do not like it at all. This chapter is about physical activity, which for you, may or may not include sport. The important thing is to find an activity you enjoy doing so that you gain pleasure from it and want to keep doing it. To gain all the benefits of exercise, it needs to be sufficiently taxing to increase your heart rate and breathing, as well as working major muscle groups. A gentle stroll may be pleasant but a truly brisk walk will do a lot more good. Apart from all the competitive team sports, beneficial exercise can include: running; cycling; walking; climbing; rambling; dancing; gardening; skateboarding; ice skating; skiing; surfing; judo; gymnastics; aerobics; rowing; canoeing; weight lifting; and tennis to name but a few. Of course, you can always get exercise in your own home. Performing press-ups, sit-ups and walking briskly up and down the stairs ten times, will all turn your home into a gym without the need for any equipment. There is always a way to fit exercise into our lives; we just need to decide we are going to do it and the prospect of better physical and mental health sounds like a powerful motivation to me.

Summary
- We evolved large brains partly because of all the exercise our ancestors took.
- Exercise helps to reduce depression and anxiety, especially when performed in green spaces.
- Regular activity improves memory and reduces the chance of dementia.
- Exercise improves our strength, stamina, balance and cardiovascular system.
- Our bones become stronger with weight-bearing activity.
- Exercise improves our sleep and increases our insulin sensitivity, both of which reduce the chance of metabolic diseases.
- Exercise is vital for our physical and mental health.

Chapter 13

SUNSHINE AND SLEEP

Have you ever wondered why the human race has people with white skin and people with black skin? We evolved in Africa and, as we lost our body hair to improve our ability to sweat, it would be logical to assume that our most distant ancestors had black skin. We all know that skin pigmentation protects us from receiving too much ultra-violet light from the sun's rays, so why do we not all have black skin? After all, we are always told to protect ourselves from the sun's harmful radiation. People living on the equator have black or darker skin tones but people who originated from latitudes far from the equator, like Britain, have much lighter skin. People in between the extremes have skin colour which is lighter or darker, depending on how intensely the sun shines down on them. Evolution has ensured that, wherever we live on this planet, we are able to absorb a reasonable amount of sunshine into our skin. Why would evolution do this, if the sun's rays are the death rays we have been led to believe? As usual, it is all about the details.

It is never a good idea to let the sun burn our skin. We can do permanent damage if we let it get too red or blistered. Too much sun exposure can lead to wrinkles, premature skin ageing, pre-cancerous rough patches called keratoses and non-melanoma skin cancers. However, too little exposure to sunshine means we miss out on all the benefits that evolution wanted us to have when it took the pigment out of our skin, as we moved further north, or south.

Mood

Have you ever heard people saying that sunshine makes them feel better? We do not feel that way simply because it is not raining; we feel good because sunshine improves our biochemistry. When the bright light of sunshine enters our eyes it travels to a structure in the brain called the pineal gland. The pineal gland is responsible for the production of melatonin, which is the hormone that helps us to fall asleep. Bright light switches off melatonin, which makes us feel more alert. But more importantly, when melatonin levels go down, serotonin levels go up. Serotonin is the happiness molecule which is well-known for improving our mood. Being outside in the sunshine literally makes us feel better.

There is a condition called Seasonal Affective Disorder, or SAD. The term was coined by Dr. Norman Rosenthal, of Georgetown University, to describe the so-called winter blues: that feeling of lethargy and sadness that comes during winter's short, dull days and long, dark nights. Some people have speculated that our modern lifestyle, which keeps people indoors under artificial light for so many hours, may be encouraging a form of SAD all year round.

Rosenthal discovered that not everyone is affected badly by a lack of sunlight but for the people who are, a daily dose of bright light from a lamp, in the frequency of natural sunlight, can help to elevate mood and relieve depressive systems. Studies of shift workers also support the positive role that exposure to sunlight has on mood. Mixing up the normal light and dark cycles, by sleeping during the day and being awake at night, can disrupt the body's metabolism. Sadly, the effects can be profound for people forced to work night shifts. The disruption can negatively impact mood, weight, energy and more. People who consistently work night shifts, for example, tend to be heavier than people who don't.

Bright light is not the only mechanism by which sunshine makes us feel better. When ultraviolet light strikes our skin it stimulates the production of endorphins, which are also produced by exercise. These are molecules known as peptides and they stimulate the body's opioid system, giving rise to feelings of happiness, pain relief and stress reduction.[1]

Heart disease
As we know, high blood pressure is a risk factor for heart disease. Not so well known is the fact that we all have stores of nitric oxide in our skin. Sunshine activates these stores allowing nitric oxide to

enter the blood stream, where it relaxes blood vessel walls, causing a fall in blood pressure. Researchers at Southampton and Edinburgh Universities measured a 'significant fall in blood pressure' when volunteers were subjected to ultraviolet light.[2] The NHS tells us to reduce salt for the sake of our blood pressure, although salt reduction has a minor effect. The authorities also tell us to limit sun exposure, although it has a significant effect on lowering blood pressure.

Vitamin D

Vitamin D is known as the sunshine vitamin because it is created in our skin when the sun shines on bare flesh. (As I have mentioned before, it is made from a cholesterol molecule, so having low cholesterol could lead to low levels of vitamin D.) The need to create adequate levels of vitamin D, from sunshine, is the reason our species has white-skinned people in latitudes with much less sunshine than there is at the equator. Darker pigmentation prevents the absorption of too much solar radiation but it allows enough ultraviolet light through to produce vitamin D. In areas with little sunshine, we need to reduce pigmentation to create the same amount of this essential vitamin.

When I was at school we were taught that vitamin D is necessary for the production and maintenance of strong teeth and bones. This is always the first benefit to be mentioned when vitamin D is discussed. Whilst this is true, we have discovered that it has many more functions in our body and our knowledge of other benefits continues to grow. There are vitamin D receptors all over our bodies: in our brains and in the cells of our immune system. Evolution would not have bothered to take pigment out of our skins if vitamin D was not incredibly important.

Vitamin D is the only vitamin we can make for ourselves; all the others have to be eaten in our food. Some foods, like fatty fish, beef liver, cheese and eggs are a good natural source of vitamin D and it is also available as a supplement. It is fat soluble and therefore needs adequate fat in the diet to be absorbed. One of its jobs is to absorb calcium and phosphorus from our food and deposit it in our bones and teeth.

An organisation called the Vitamin D Council has a website with an extensive collection of research papers about the benefits of this vitamin on a vast range of human ailments. Vitamin D's ability to reduce the risk of osteoporosis and rickets is well known because these problems are caused by a lack of bone density. However, there is evidence of its protective benefits in a wide range of cancers, skin conditions like acne and eczema, heart disease, diabetes, mental health issues like depression, Alzheimer's disease and Parkinson's disease. For most of these conditions, vitamin D does not provide a complete cure or total prevention, but the research clearly shows that the higher a person's vitamin D level, the better they do when they have these problems and the less likely they are to develop them in the first place. Let us look at a few examples.

Immunity

It has been known for many years that an optimum level of Vitamin D greatly reduces the severity of respiratory infections and is a vital component of our natural, or innate, immune system. Vitamin D is produced by sunshine on the skin. Our levels, therefore, are invariably lowest during winter, which explains why influenza is so much more prevalent in the darkest months. During the Coronavirus pandemic of 2020, it was clear that certain people suffered far more than others. The elderly, and those with pre-existing metabolic diseases, either died or needed intensive care in hospital at a rate considerably higher than younger, healthy people.

In the UK, and many other countries, the authorities acted as if everybody was at equal risk despite all the evidence to the contrary. However, some researchers tested Covid-19 patients for their levels of Vitamin D, when they were admitted to hospital. An Indonesian study [3] found a death rate of only 4% among people with normal levels. People with insufficient levels of Vitamin D died at a rate of 87.8% and those who were deemed deficient in Vitamin D died from the virus at the extraordinary rate of 98.9%. A study in American hospitals by Dr Eric Hermstad showed that death or serious illness invariably occurred among those with

Vitamin D levels below 25 nanograms (ng) per ml, which is 5ng/ml below their national average of 30ng/ml. None of the patients admitted to hospital had a Vitamin D level above 40ng/ml, suggesting that this prevented hospitalisation. Why did the UK Government's scientific advisers fail to tell us all about these findings?

Between 70 and 80% of people infected with this coronavirus had either mild symptoms, or no symptoms at all. A combination of good health and a robust immune system was all the protection we needed from a virus which was predicted, by computer models, to kill half a million people in the UK. The great majority of deaths occurred in hospitals and care homes where people are generally in poor health, are fed an imperfect diet and rarely, if ever, go outside in the sunshine.

Autism

Around 700,000 people in the UK have some form of autism, which is just over 1% of the population. The prevalence has increased five-fold since 1990 and that is a major concern. Children with autism have difficulty communicating. They have trouble understanding what other people think and feel, making it very hard for them to express themselves, either with words or through gestures. We refer to an autistic spectrum because the social impairment of autistic people can vary from mild to severely debilitating.

Research has shown a strong link between young children with autism and a low level of vitamin D in the mother during pregnancy.[4] This implies that vitamin D is essential for the development of the areas of the brain involved in communication. Autistic children are invariably found to have low levels of vitamin D themselves. A study of 4,229 women found those with the lowest levels of vitamin D in mid-pregnancy, and at the time of the birth, had children with twice the risk of autistic traits. The maternal vitamin D deficiency is not the only factor that increases autism risk. A 2018 study of 3-year-olds found those children in the lowest 25% of vitamin D levels had a massive 260% increased risk of autism. Pregnant women and new mothers need to be made more aware of the vital importance of an excellent diet, in addition to exposure to some sunshine, during pregnancy.

The UK's National Autistic Society claims that autism is incurable. However, Dr John Cannell has published scientific papers showing otherwise. In a published trial of vitamin D in autism, which Dr Cannell co-authored, 83 autistic children completed 3 months of a daily, high-dose vitamin D treatment (5,000 IU/day). Eighty per cent of the children who received the vitamin D had significantly improved outcomes, mainly in the sections of standard tests that measure behaviour, eye contact and attention span. A case report in the influential journal, *Pediatrics*, found that high-dose, vitamin D supplementation remarkably reduced the core symptoms of autism in a 32-month-old toddler.

Colorectal cancer

This is the type of cancer that the World Health Organisation wants you to believe is not only caused by eating processed meat but is also possibly caused by eating fresh, red meat. The information they used came from observational studies and I have explained how unreliable these can be. However, sometimes they are the only research available and, therefore, I feel justified in quoting a paper published in the journal, *Cancer Prevention Research*, in 2011. The researchers did an analysis of eight previous studies and they published their results under the title, '*Circulating levels of vitamin D and colon and rectal cancer.*' They discovered that people with the highest levels of vitamin D in their body had a 50% lower chance of developing rectal cancer, and a 23% lower chance of developing colon cancer than people with the lowest levels of vitamin D. This does not prove that vitamin D prevents colorectal cancer, but the WHO claimed meat was causing this cancer, quoting results that showed an 18% increase in risk. It appears from this research that low levels of vitamin D are clearly more dangerous than the consumption of red meat when it comes to colorectal cancer. Why did the WHO omit to tell us this piece of information when it scared everybody away from eating one of the most nutritious foods available?

Multiple sclerosis

Multiple sclerosis is a debilitating condition where the body's immune system attacks the nerves in the brain and spinal cord. Because these nerves provide messages to so many different areas of the body, the symptoms of multiple sclerosis can affect a whole range of functions. Sufferers experience problems walking, talking, speaking, swallowing and sometimes even thinking. It affects women more than men and usually starts between 20 to 40 years of age.

Nobody is certain of the cause of multiple sclerosis but it is more common across the world in areas far from the equator and in people born in early spring. This suggests that there may be a link between the amount of sunshine people get and the likelihood of developing this awful disease. Research has shown that when immune system cells are exposed to vitamin D, in laboratory experiments, they become less inflamed. This could mean that vitamin D offers some protection to our immune system and makes it less likely to attack other cells in our body.

An interesting observation has been reported by a couple of Oxford University scientists. The incidence of multiple sclerosis shot up almost 700% in Tehran from 1989 to 2005. What could have caused this? Ten years earlier, in 1979, the Iranian Revolution had brought in strict codes of dress for women, which included head scarves and almost total body coverage. Did the avoidance of sunshine on Iranian skin cause this huge spike in the disease?[5]

Melanoma

There are three types of skin cancer: basal cell carcinoma; squamous cell carcinoma; and melanoma. The first two are fairly common and easily treated. Melanoma, however, is a very aggressive cancer with low survival rates and an incidence which has more than doubled since the 1980s. The NHS and other authorities tell us that melanoma is caused by exposure to sunshine but that is not entirely correct. People who have had severe sunburn in the past are more likely to get melanoma than people who have never burnt their skin but statistics clearly show that office workers get more melanoma than people who work outside. How do we explain that?

Unhealthy exposure to the sun can cause sunburn resulting in damage to the skin cells and their DNA. It also damages the melanocytes which produce melanin, the pigment in our skin. Melanoma starts as cancer of these melanocytes but it can then spread throughout the body. Healthy sun exposure produces vitamin D, which has a protective action against cancer cells. Sunshine also builds a resistance to the effects of ultraviolet light by gradually increasing the melanin levels, or creating a slight tan.

Melanoma is more common among people living far from the equator. If it was caused simply by sun exposure that fact could not be true.[6] The people most likely to succumb are white-skinned people who sunbathe for long periods each day on their once-a-year summer holiday. They get excessive exposure on skin that is not ready for it. The sun's beneficial and harmful effects are caused by different wavelengths of ultraviolet light. UVB produces vitamin D and stimulates the tanning process. UVA is the wavelength that causes all the damage. Unfortunately, UVB is easier to block than UVA. We should never sunbathe behind glass because UVB is filtered out by glass but UVA can pass right through. Even the earth's atmosphere can reduce UVB; evening and morning sun has less UVB than midday sun. It sounds counterintuitive but it is best to expose our skin to the sun in the middle of the day to maximise the benefits. Healthy sun exposure consists of uncovering as much skin as modesty and decency will allow, in the middle of the day for between 10 and 15 minutes, without any sun cream.

Almost everybody is aware of the dangers of sunburn, and the campaigns to persuade us all to either hide from the sun or cover ourselves in factor 30; advice followed by the majority of people. According to the *American Academy of Dermatology*, the incidence of malignant melanoma skin cancer, in most developed countries, has risen faster than any other cancer type since the mid-1950s. If we are all protecting ourselves more than we did 65 years ago, how come melanoma is increasing?

What else has changed dramatically over recent decades? The answer to that question, of course, is our diet. Specifically, a decrease in saturated fat and a huge increase in polyunsaturated seed oils containing a high ratio of omega 6 fatty acids. Lipid molecules compete with each other to form cell membranes and a high intake of omega 6 in the diet causes a high percentage of omega 6 in skin cell membranes. As discussed in Chapter 8, polyunsaturated fats are highly reactive and easily oxidised and omega 6 increases inflammation. The energy in UVA is the perfect catalyst to oxidise these cell membranes and increase the inflammatory effects of omega 6, both of which increase the chance of cancer growth. Cell membranes, when made predominantly of saturated fat, are much less reactive and are better able to resist the effects of UVA. The most effective thing any of us can do to reduce our chance of melanoma is to eliminate so-called vegetable oils from our diet. Unfortunately, they are in almost every processed food on the supermarket shelf.

Sources of vitamin D
While sunshine is the best way to maintain good vitamin D levels, it is impossible to get enough sunshine during the winter months in countries like Britain. Therefore, we need to be aware of the best food sources from which we can obtain a plentiful supply. These are oily fish like salmon, herring, mackerel, sardines, oysters, shrimp and tuna. Beef liver is an excellent source and so are eggs. Red meat, milk and milk products, like cheese and yoghurt, have some vitamin D too. All these animal sources contain vitamin D3 which is the type our bodies need. Plant sources of vitamin D are rare and, where it does occur, it is in the form of D2. Studies have shown that D2 has less than one third of the potency of vitamin D3.[7]

The vegan claim that a plant-based diet is more healthy than one containing animal foods cannot possibly be true. If I have not yet convinced you of the importance of this vitamin, perhaps the words of Professor Holick will help. Michael Holick is Professor of Medicine, Physiology and Biophysics at Boston University and he says, "Vitamin D deficiency is a global pandemic that has serious health consequences for children and adults. Improvement in the world's vitamin D status could significantly reduce the risk of many chronic illnesses including cardiovascular diseases, type 2 diabetes and many deadly cancers as well as infectious diseases including upper respiratory tract infections, influenza and tuberculosis."

What do the authorities tell us to do? Their advice includes: avoid sunshine or apply lots of sunscreen; swap saturated fat for vegetable oils; eat a low fat diet; eat lots of fruit and vegetables; and cut back on meat and animal foods. It should be no surprise there is a pandemic of vitamin D deficiency and an escalation of cancers and auto-immune diseases.

The importance of sleep

We all have some knowledge of the relationship between sleep and our ability to function throughout the day. I expect everyone has experienced the fatigue, bad mood and lack of focus that can follow a night of poor sleep, but I wonder how many people realise that a lack of sleep, especially on a regular basis, is associated with long-term ill health? A chronic lack of quality sleep is linked to an increased risk of diabetes, high blood pressure, heart disease, depression and obesity and, of course, these conditions can shorten our lives.

Why am I talking about sleep in a chapter on sunshine? Our ability to sleep well depends on the hormone melatonin, produced by the pineal gland. Melatonin helps us to go to sleep and its production is increased by the onset of darkness and the cycle of our circadian rhythm. Bright light in the morning helps to set our internal clock; therefore, exposure to sunshine, early in the day, helps us to sleep better at night. Conversely, bright light in the evening reduces melatonin and makes it harder to fall asleep. Computer screens and smart phones emit blue light which is particularly damaging to melatonin production. Reading a book before bedtime can help us to feel drowsy but looking at a screen can have the opposite effect.

Children, whose development is dependent on good quality sleep, should avoid having computers, televisions or smart phones in their bedrooms. There has been a big increase in referrals of children to sleep specialists in recent years, and many of these problems are caused by electronic devices in bedrooms. If you are a parent of a child, it is very important to provide an environment suitable for your child to obtain the sleep that is essential for their health and development. Letting them have a phone or tablet in their bedroom at night is not a good idea because it can lead to several problems in the future.

During sleep our bodies secrete hormones that help to control appetite, energy metabolism and glucose processing. Too little sleep upsets the balance of these and other hormones. Poor sleep leads to an increase in the production of the stress hormone, cortisol, which in turn decreases the ability of insulin to do its job correctly. Insufficient sleep is also associated with lower levels of leptin, the hormone that tells the brain that it has had enough food, as well as producing higher levels of ghrelin, the hormone that stimulates appetite. As a result, people who sleep badly are more likely to overeat. One third of children leave primary school severely overweight. While too much carbohydrate is the primary cause, too little sleep is certain to have a significant influence. Also, several studies have shown that adults who are regularly sleeping less than five hours per night have a greatly increased risk of developing diabetes.[8]

A single sleepless night can make people irritable and moody the following day, so it is not a surprise to learn that chronic sleep loss may lead to long-term mood disorders. Long-term sleep problems have been linked to depression, anxiety and mental distress. In one study, people who slept for only four and a half hours per night reported feeling more stressed, sad, angry, and mentally exhausted. In another study, they showed declining levels of optimism and sociability. All of these symptoms improved dramatically when the subjects returned to a normal sleep schedule.

A lack of sleep is not only bad for our health, it can also be dangerous for us and others. Sleep-deprived people are much more likely to make mistakes and cause accidents. A lot of road traffic collisions are thought to be caused by tiredness. Medical errors in hospitals are frequently the result of junior doctors being forced to work ridiculously long hours without the chance for sleep. Investigators have concluded that the nuclear disasters at both Three Mile Island and Chernobyl were caused by a lack of sleep among staff making critical decisions.[9]

Concentration, working memory, mathematical ability, and logical reasoning are all aspects of brain function which can be compromised by sleep deprivation. However, not all of these functions rely on the same regions of the brain, nor are they impacted by sleep deprivation to the same degree. For example, the prefrontal cortex is responsible for many high-level, cognitive functions and is particularly vulnerable to a lack of sleep. Consequently, people who are sleep deprived will perform badly in tasks that require logical reasoning or complex thought. This is really important for students who make the mistake of cramming for exams by staying up all night to revise. Not only can their brains not function properly, but it is during sleep that long term memories are created. If you revise all night instead of sleeping, you diminish the amount of information you can retain, thus reducing your ability to think clearly. If you stay awake with the help of caffeine and sugary 'energy' drinks, you risk compounding the problem. A small dose of caffeine can help you to concentrate for a short period of time but large doses, taken over many hours, can cause anxiety, panic, reduced attention and ineffective memory. This is not what you want during an important exam.

Insomnia

A lot of people have difficulty either getting to sleep or staying asleep and this makes them feel tired and irritable the next day. Figures suggest that 1 in every 10 adults is taking some sort of sleeping tablet to get them through the night, and this is costing the NHS about £50 million per year. Medication can be useful to help people get back into the routine of regular sleep but tablets are usually of benefit only if they are taken for a short period of time. Long-term use leads to tolerance which means we have to take a stronger dose to achieve the same effect, and this leads to an accumulation of side effects.

A sleep routine is usually the best way to improve our ability to enjoy a good night's sleep. The most effective things we can do include the following:

1. Exposure to bright light in the morning, especially sunshine if it is available.

2. Exercise each day, but not too close to bedtime. Outdoor exercise in green spaces is best because it improves our mood and reduces stress.

3. Try to go to bed and get up each day at the same time. Our circadian rhythms help us to sleep and they love a regular routine.

4. Avoid caffeine in the late afternoon and evening. The stimulant effect of caffeine lasts for hours and can stop us falling asleep.

5. Reduce alcohol intake. Alcohol makes us drowsy and can help us to fall asleep but it is fairly quickly metabolised and the sedative effect often wears off in the middle of the night, causing us to wake far too early.

6. Bedrooms should be dark, quiet and cool. Have warm bedcovers rather than a warm bedroom.

7. Avoid bright lights, including electronic screens, in the hour before bedtime.

8. Do not eat a large meal close to bedtime. A full stomach makes it harder to nod off.

9. A warm bath or shower before bed can help because we cool down afterwards and a falling temperature is one of the triggers for sleep.

10. If you are worried or stressed and have a lot on your mind, it will be harder to fall asleep. Try to put them out of your mind with the help of soothing music or an interesting book.

11. Whatever you do, do not worry about all the terrible things I have suggested can happen to you if you don't get enough sleep!

Summary:

- Exposure to a certain amount of sunshine is essential for our health. It creates vitamin D, improves our mood and reduces blood pressure.
- Vitamin D does far more than create strong bones and teeth. It protects us from a wide range of ailments including autism, cancer and multiple sclerosis.
- The bright light of sunshine helps to set our circadian rhythms, which in turn help us to sleep. Adequate sleep is an essential component of good health.

Chapter 14

FIT CHILDREN FINISH FIRST IN THE CLASSROOM

In today's politically correct world, you are unlikely to hear anybody in public office saying, 'Physically fit children are academically superior to unfit children', which is a problem because research from around the world has proved this to be true. As I explained in Chapter 3, physical activity increases the production of nerve-growth factors in the brain. One of the reasons we possess elaborate brains is because our ancestors, over a long period of time, were chasing animals for food. It has recently been discovered that the process of enhancing brain function by exercise produces rapid results in the development of children.

In October 2013 Professor John Reilly, from Strathclyde University, and Doctor Josie Booth, from Dundee University, published their findings from a study which is following the lives of 5,000 children born in 1991 and 1992. This group is known as the 'Avon Cohort'. The researchers examined the amount of moderate to vigorous physical activity the children were doing at the age of 11 and compared this to their academic performance in English, mathematics and science. Their results showed that the children with higher levels of moderate to vigorous exercise had better academic performance across all three subjects, and this was true for both boys and girls. The children were assessed again at both 13 and 15 years of age, when it was found that their academic achievement was still linked to how much energetic exercise they had taken when they were 11.

Lesley Cottrell is a professor of children's health at West Virginia University, and in 2010 she published the results of a study into the link between children's physical fitness and academic performance.[1] She analysed the body mass index, fitness levels and academic test scores of 725 ten-year-old students. The research focussed on the children's fitness level, rather than their weight. She then compared that information to the same students' physical fitness and academic performance two years later.

Cottrell found that the children with the best average scores in reading, maths, science and social studies were physically fit at the start and at the end of the study. The next best group academically, in all four subjects, was made up of children who were not fit when they were 10 but had become fit by the time of the re-test. The children who had lost their fitness levels between 10 and 12 years of age were third in academic performance, and children who were never physically fit, during either test, had the lowest academic performance.

The difference between the academic performance of fit children and unfit children has been shown in other studies. However, this is one of the first to show that losing physical fitness, over a two-year period, also lowers test scores and that improving fitness over the same time scale improves academic results.

Professor Mark Mon-Williams and PhD student, Liam Hill, ran a two-week trial in six primary schools in Aberdeen, which involved 1,224 children aged between 8 and 11 years old.[2] During the first week, half of the group received a teacher-led programme of physical exercise, which lasted 15 minutes and took place in the classroom about 30 minutes after lunch; the other half of the children did no exercise. In the second week the two groups swapped their exercise or no-exercise routines. At the end of each school day all the children completed one of five psychometric tests, so that each test was delivered once after exercise and once after no exercise. Fifteen minutes of exercise for just five days is a small change to make during a child's school day, but the results showed a significant improvement in test scores among the children doing the physical exercises.

The majority of this type of research has been done in America. In 2012 Michigan State University tested 312 eight-year-olds for all-round fitness by measuring their body fat, muscle strength, flexibility and endurance. They then compared that to the children's grades and test scores throughout the school year. The results showed that the fittest children got the highest test scores, regardless of whether they were boys or girls.

Professor Petri, from the University of North Texas, studied 1,211 children of very diverse ethnic and social backgrounds. As well as testing their fitness and academic achievement, he also took into account other influences like self-esteem, social support and economic status. At the end of the study he said, "Cardiorespiratory fitness was the only factor that we consistently found to have a positive effect on both boys' and girls' grades in reading and maths tests." So, the frequently quoted idea that children from poor families, given little support, are always going to struggle in school because of their backgrounds is not proven in this study.[3] In fact, physical fitness was shown to be the most important factor relating to academic grades.

There are many similar studies, by different universities, which also found a direct link between physical fitness and performance in school, but at the University of Michigan they went a step further and showed why this happens. Professor Art Kramer studied a group of nine and ten-year-olds by testing their ability to use oxygen while running on a treadmill. This is a standard measure of fitness, which is often used by athletes, and he discovered that the physically fit children were much more efficient at using oxygen than the less-fit children. When he tested their mental capabilities, it was clear that the fit children had a greater ability to remember and integrate various types of information than their less-fit peers. He knew that a part of the brain called the hippocampus is particularly important for the formation of memories, so he gave these children an electronic brain scan to measure the relative size of structures in the brain. When he analysed the MRI (magnetic resonance imaging) data, he found that the physically fit children had a bigger hippocampus than the out-of-shape ones. On average, it was 12% larger which is clear evidence that physically fit children perform better in academic tests than unfit children. This happens because the physical exercise, which has made them fit, has also enlarged the parts of the brain that improve memory through the production of nerve growth factors.

We have already looked at why evolution has given us the best brains on the planet, and why exercise was crucial to that process. Evolution takes a very long time but this recent research shows that the beneficial effects of exercise on the brain operate over much shorter timescales. Those children in Michigan were only ten years old but the energetically active ones had a hippocampus 12% bigger than their inactive friends, and the children in Aberdeen showed improvements after only 15 minutes of activity.

It is clear from the evidence that fitter children do better in school than unfit children, but how fit, on average, are children in the UK?

According to Dr Gavin Sandercock, from the Centre for Sports and Exercise Science at the University of Essex, youngsters in Britain today are significantly less fit than they were two decades ago. He and his fellow researchers tested 300 ten-year-olds from an affluent area in Chelmsford in 1998, and then repeated the tests with another 300 ten-year-olds from the same area in 2008. They used shuttle runs to test cardiovascular fitness, which is a measure of how efficiently the heart and lungs deliver oxygen to muscle tissue to aid endurance and prolong physical activity. The results were shocking. The fitness level of girls had declined by 7% and boys had fallen back by 9% in a decade. Even the slim children were significantly less fit. Dr Sandercock blames our less active lifestyles:

"Children are not doing as many physical activities as before. They are using their spare time to play more computer games, more time watching television, or more time online. They don't climb trees any more, they don't use their bikes any more. I read last week that Britain is highly up-to-date with technology, with more computers-per-household than anywhere else in Europe, but that means our children are playing on computers more. The drop in fitness is very, very large."

Sixty minutes of exercise per day is the internationally accepted and recommended standard for children's activity, but when the exercise levels of the 'Avon Cohort' were tested, the average for boys was only 29 minutes and for girls it was a paltry

18 minutes. Fewer than 1% of the children were doing the recommended hour per day.

Our Government is well aware of this terrible state of affairs but what is it doing about it? It is doing what governments always do, which is spending tax payers' money. Over recent years the Government has spent more than £1.5 billion on schemes to encourage more sport in schools. They have also invested £75 million in their flagship 'Change For Life' programme, which is meant to encourage healthier, more active lifestyles, and is particularly targeted at children. It would appear not to be working very well.

Children spend a great deal of their lives in school and the main purpose of school is to acquire knowledge by learning. The scientific evidence we have seen shows clearly that physical fitness is essential to successful learning; therefore, schools should be making sure that their students are physically active and fit. How well do they do this?

Schools in the UK are required to give their children two hours of physical education each week up to the age of 16, but what does the PE curriculum say they should do during those two hours? The entire primary school PE curriculum is available on the Department for Education's website, and it gives the clear impression that physical education is another subject to be taught like geography or history. This is a copy of the introduction to the curriculum:

"During Key Stage 1 pupils build on their natural enthusiasm for movement, using it to explore and learn about their world. They start to work and play with other pupils in pairs and small groups. By watching, listening and experimenting, they develop their skills in movement and coordination, and enjoy expressing and testing themselves in a variety of situations."

The curriculum then goes into more detail:

Pupils should be taught to:
- *explore how to choose and apply skills and actions in sequence and in combination*
- *vary the way they perform skills by using simple tactics and movement phrases*

- *apply rules and conventions for different activities*
- *describe what they have done*
- *observe, describe and copy what others have done*
- *use what they have learnt to improve the quality of their work*
- *know how important it is to be active*
- *to describe how their bodies feel during different activities.*

The pupils learn all these skills through the following activities: dance; games; gymnastics; swimming and water-safety. The curriculum then suggests ways in which the various activities can be cross-referenced to other subjects like science, music and information technology. Under the latter it suggests, "Pupils could use videos of movements and actions to develop their ideas."

Like all other subjects, the children need to be assessed for their competence in PE and each child is awarded a level between one and nine. The difference between each level is small but all of them refer to such concepts as:

"When performing, they draw on what they know about strategy, tactics and composition. They analyse and comment on skills and techniques. They explain why regular, safe exercise is good for their fitness and health."

I am sure that good PE teachers do their best to get their children physically active, but throughout the entire PE curriculum, there is absolutely no mention of a raised heart rate. There is no requirement to test a child's physical fitness. There is no requirement to improve a child's physical fitness. I am going to repeat that: in the PE curriculum there is no requirement to improve a child's physical fitness!

If I can find all this information linking academic attainment to physical fitness, surely the Department for Education could find it too? All government departments have scientific advisers and I looked up the Chief Scientific adviser to the Education Department. According to the gov.uk website in March 2019, the post is held by Dr Tim Leunig. I imagined that he would be a specialist in child development, or brain development or at least education. It turns out that he is not a scientist at all: he is an economist. Why has the Department for Education appointed a scientific adviser without any knowledge of relevant science?

Adults benefit too

To ensure there is no doubt about the link between physical fitness and academic achievement, we should look at what they discovered in Sweden. The study involved 1.2 million Swedish men doing military service, who were born between 1950 and 1976. The research group analysed the results of both physical tests and IQ tests when the men enrolled. The study shows a clear link between good physical fitness and better results for the IQ test.[4] The strongest links are for logical thinking and verbal comprehension.

"Being fit means that you also have good heart and lung capacity and that your brain gets plenty of oxygen," says Michael Nilsson, professor at the Sahlgrenska Academy and chief physician at the University Hospital. "We are also seeing that there are nerve growth factors that are important. This may be one of the reasons why we can see a clear link between physical fitness and intelligence." By analysing data for twins, the researchers have been able to determine that it is primarily environmental factors and not genetics that explain the link between fitness and a higher IQ.

"We have also shown that those youngsters who improve their physical fitness between the ages of 15 and 18 increase their cognitive performance," says Maria Åberg, who is also a researcher and physician. "This being the case, physical education is a subject that has an important place in schools, and is an absolute must if we want to do well in maths and other theoretical subjects." The researchers have also compared the results from fitness tests during national service with the socio-economic status of the men later in life. Those who were fit at 18 were more likely to go into higher education, and many secured more qualified jobs.

Sport or fitness?

The researchers in all of these studies have stated that their results show how important it is to prioritise physical education in schools. But it turns out that physical education in British schools does not even try to improve a child's physical fitness; they concentrate on skills, techniques and learning to explain why exercise is good for you.

The current school curriculum for England and Wales was introduced in 2014. At the same time, the authorities announced that they intended to increase their focus on competitive sport. The reason for this approach appears to be a mixture of widely-held views that we all need to be competitive in a competitive world and that sport 'builds character'. They also want to ensure that schools are able to identify and nurture Britain's talented athletes of the future.

There is, perhaps, also a reaction against the absurd idea of non-competitive sports day. Sports day ought to be a celebration of physical achievement. To take the competition out of it is the same, in principle, as holding uncompetitive exams, where everybody gets the same mark no matter what they have written. Somebody with a talent for athletics should be able to explore and test their abilities in the same way that somebody with a talent for mathematics can do in the classroom.

My personal preferences are irrelevant to the information in this book; however, I am going to mention them to emphasise the point I am about to make. I am a huge fan of competitive sport. I spent twenty years of my life as a competitive athlete and I still enjoy the excitement generated by live sport. My sporting career began with school sport and then progressed to a local club. This is how nearly everyone who goes on to represent Great Britain begins their journey. I do not ever want to see competitive sport removed from schools. However, I do not believe for one moment that an exclusive emphasis on competitive sport is the best way to get all school children to enjoy and participate in the sort of life-long, energetic activity that is essential to their physical, mental and emotional well-being. I am not alone in this opinion.

A comprehensive review, published by the Young Foundation in September 2012, said that the government's insistence on competitive team sports will 'alienate schoolchildren' instead of tackling their sedentary lifestyles. It pointed out that "an epidemic of inactivity among all age groups is costing the UK £8.2 billion a year" and that "the emphasis on traditional, competitive team-based sports is out of line with the way many young people want to participate."

Will Norman, co-author of the report and the think-tank's director of research, said: "Kids want to do much more informal sports like street running, parkour and Zumba-type activities that are very flexible, can be done wearing different types of clothing or while listening to music and can be done individually. Competitive sports will work for some people. But if we want to get the most inactive children to be active, we need to change our thinking. We need a philosophy that's driven by the people we are trying to target and not provide things that the most inactive don't want to do."

Other reports have shown that over 50% of girls dislike PE and many of them are so alienated by it that they are put off any type of physical activity for life. I think everybody already knew that some people enjoy competitive sport while other people do not. The Young Foundation's research has shown that many of the children who are alienated by competitive sport are keen to be active, if they are doing something they enjoy. This is very important information that the government appears to be ignoring, judging by their response to the report:

"We want more young people to take part in competitive sport, not only so they lead healthy and active lifestyles but also so they develop new skills and learn how to work as a team. That is why we are putting competitive sport at the heart of the new primary school curriculum and extending school games."

I have done a lot of research for this book, however, I cannot find any conclusive evidence for the benefits of competitive sport over other types of physical activity in the development of young people. All the evidence from around the world is clear: children who are physically fit do better in school and in later life than children who are unfit. Fit children grow into fit adults. The Swedish study of 1.2 million men showed that the fit ones had higher IQs and got better jobs. Surely that is the outcome we all want from the time children spend in school?

Summary:

- Physical activity increases the production of nerve-growth chemicals in the brain, improving memory and connectivity.
- Children in the UK are becoming increasingly unfit because they spend less time outdoors than children from the past.
- The PE curriculum has no requirement to improve a child's fitness and competitive sport alienates some children from the joys of exercise.

Chapter 15

PLAYTIME MAKES US BETTER PEOPLE

It is a universal truth that children love to play and every child around the world is born with a strong instinct to do so. True play is spontaneous and can take many different forms but, above all, it comes from within the child. Sometimes play is solitary and sometimes it takes place in groups. It can involve real or imaginary toys. It brings huge joy to children of all ages but it is never truly playful unless a child is free to join or leave the activity at any time, nor if the play is directed by an adult.

Children are not the only youngsters to play. Most mammals, and even some birds, have the same instinct and need. Frolicking puppies and kittens may spring to mind but it is also known that the young of meerkats, lions, ravens, coyotes, elephants and even rats have strong instincts to play. When such a diverse range of creatures all have the same need, surely there must be a strong evolutionary reason for it, but what is that need? As long ago as 1898 the German naturalist, Karl Gros, published his book *The Play of Animals* in which he proposed that play was a rehearsal for the challenges of life. He had observed that predatory animals tend to play games involving pouncing and fighting, while animals that are preyed upon often play running and evading games. His idea that play is a way of learning has become generally accepted, despite the inability of researchers to prove this is true.[1]

Dr Jaak Panksepp is a neuroscientist who specialises in studying the emotion of animals. When he allowed young laboratory rats to play with each other, they would chase, fight, roll over and make a chirping sound, which they did not make at other times. He had no idea what this sound was until it occurred to him that it might be laughter. He flipped some of these young rats onto their backs and tickled their abdomens, noting that they all produced the same chirping sound they made when playing. People who regard rats as dirty, sewer-living vermin, may find it hard to believe that young rats play with each other and laugh when they do so, but it is true. This information reinforces the fact that play, and the enjoyment of play, is a very widespread and deep-seated evolutionary process.

Dr Panksepp points out that the physical structure of a human brain shows clear evidence of three evolutionary layers. The part of our brain which evolved first produces our instincts and emotions. These basic feelings and actions happen without conscious thought and, when they occur in a young brain, they create new links and pathways to the next layer. This second level of brain development involves learning and memory. The desire to play, for example, is a basic, instinctive process; however, the playing of games is a secondary process because games have structure and therefore need memory. Many creatures have the first two layers of brain structure but highly developed animals, like ourselves, have a third layer which is found in the neocortex. The memories in the second layer create links and pathways to the third layer, which is where the more complicated processes of thought, imagination, planning and decision-making occur. Therefore, how we control our basic instincts is dependent upon the pathways we create in our brain between our instincts and our memories and between memories and new thoughts. In the *American Journal of Play,* Panksepp wrote:

The human genome does not contain enough information to construct a fully social brain. Play, and the many other basic emotional systems of ancient regions of the brain, are the tools that allow the social brain to develop. Realising that this is so, compels us to consider how much of the human brain is created by social learning as opposed to ancestral genetic moulding. And if most of the social brain matures under the tutelage of environmental factors, those factors can in turn help support life-long mental health or they can help create a lifetime of emotional problems. Which path a child follows in life very much depends on how we recruit, use, and invest in the social-emotional tools that nature has provided for jump-starting optimal development. [2]

Play is necessary because the brain of a young child is not, as thought by many people, a small version of an adult brain that simply needs to be filled with information. It has all the structures of an adult brain but it does not have the connections and pathways that it needs to function as a successful adult. Play creates the brain pathways which allow us to control our basic emotions. Play provides the input for young brains to develop the most important skills in life: creativity, empathy, intuition, imagination, consideration, bravery and calmness. These skills cannot be taught in school lessons but the brain is able to achieve all this because of different types of play.

Play with Adults

When a baby is born it needs to bond with the person who is caring for it and that person needs to bond with the baby. Infants can receive love from many different adults but they need to form a secure attachment with one person: usually the mother. This secure attachment bond forms the emotional relationship between a baby and mother and it is created by the responses each gives to the signals of the other, as expressed by movements, gestures, and sounds. The success of this wordless relationship enables a child to feel secure enough to develop fully, and affects how he or she will interact, communicate, and form relationships throughout life. It is developed by giving the baby plenty of attention, especially in the form of physical skin-to-skin contact, as well as eye contact. It involves caring for a child physically, through feeding and cleaning, and emotionally with love and protection.

Responding to each other through smiles and laughter produces hormones like oxytocin, which acts to strengthen the bond between parent and child. A secure attachment bond enables the parts of a baby's brain responsible for social and emotional development, communication and relationships to flourish. It is a vital influence on a child's social, emotional, intellectual and physical growth. An insecure attachment bond leads to confusion, lack of trust, learning difficulties and poor relationships in later life. Whilst feeding and changing a new-born baby are both essential, play and laughter are also very important in an infant's development.

Physical Play

Physical play encourages children to want to run, jump, chase and climb, so that they develop their physical abilities, fitness and coordination. You can see this happen whenever children reach the beach or a park after a long car journey. As soon as they are free from the confines of the car, they often start to run around, spontaneously and happily, driven by their instinct to play. This natural exuberance allows them to develop their muscular coordination, strength and balance. It improves their cardiovascular fitness and it integrates the actions of muscles, nerves and brain functions.

Physical play also involves the essential ingredients of excitement and fear. You experience both of these emotions when you are being chased in a game of tag: will you be caught or not? You feel them both when you climb a tree: will you reach that other branch or will you fall? Children enjoy this excitement and a certain amount of fear. They will naturally climb to a level which is exciting and slightly scary but they never willingly put themselves into real danger. At each stage of their physical development, they know what they are capable of. It would be cruel to make a child climb something they find truly frightening; however, it is also cruel to prevent a child from experiencing any fear. If someone never experiences fear during childhood, they may be overwhelmed with terror when they are frightened as an adult. They will be unable to cope with the unfamiliar surge of the stress hormone, cortisol, or they may be unable to distinguish between a slight risk and a severe danger.

Rough and tumble play, where children push, wrestle and fight each other, is the type of play that nearly all animals enjoy. Adults in authority often stop this kind of play because they are concerned someone might get hurt. Children, however, develop a great sense of trust when engaging like this because they know it is play and they are not really trying to hurt their playmate. When accidents do happen, and someone scrapes their knee or elbow, an important process takes place. Pain receptors are activated and developed and the injured body adapts to dealing with pain.

Recent research suggests that if someone never experiences pain during childhood, the degree of pain felt as an adult can feel excruciating.

Object Play

The curiosity that children have for all sorts of objects is a clear sign that play is a form of learning. You learn a lot about the physical world when you go from a sandpit, to building a tower of wooden blocks, and then to floating a plastic duck in the bath. Handling, feeling and experimenting with a large variety of physical things, however, is more than just learning about gravity, friction, texture and size. Playing with objects develops specific brain pathways and children who are comfortable manipulating objects and materials, also become good at manipulating words, ideas and concepts.

The scientific study of complex play involving objects, and its relation to overall ability, has prompted research into how ready people are for the challenges of work. An absence of fixing things by hand during one's childhood may well mean a deficiency in solving complex problems at work as an adult. Research has shown that manipulating objects with your hands develops the problem-solving pathways in your brain.[2] To be a good engineer, for example, may mean that the time spent building model airplanes, or constructing a den in the woods, are just as important as getting a degree. It becomes especially true if the engineer is expected to work as an innovative problem solver. This is another example of the physical world and the development of the brain working in harmony.

Fantasy Play

Imagination and creativity are stimulated by fantasy play. While dressing up as a pirate, a fairy, a firefighter or a caped crusader may appear to be mere frivolity, it encourages children to process abstract thoughts and to imagine they are something or someone else. The ability to think in the abstract, rather than just the here and now, is a function of a highly developed brain and an essential tool for adult life. The brain circuits for abstract thought are

175

allowed to flourish when a child takes a bowl, for example, turns it over and it becomes a hat, or an igloo, or a mountain with a dragon inside. The ability to treat things symbolically is wonderful training for the processing of ideas and theories and for thinking through the consequences of our actions, which are all essential adult skills. It also helps children to learn to read because there is nothing more symbolic than words on a page. The letters d, o and g do not bark or wag their tail when put together but they represent the dog that does. That concept is much easier for children to understand after they have used fantasy play to develop their brain's ability to process abstract thoughts.

The development of creativity is also a vital function of fantasy play. Creativity is not something that can be taught and research has shown that it is reduced by being tested. When students were asked to invent creatures from an alien world, they were much more creative when they were told they would not be judged on the results, compared to when they were told they would be judged. When your children are playing with a doll's house and they have everyone entering through the windows, they are developing creativity. They know that people use the door to go inside but if you 'correct' them, you risk putting a big dent in their imagination.

The success of fantasy play, within a group of children, requires a broad range of attributes which most adults would be happy to have. The process requires a high level of social skills. The children need imagination to create the game and negotiating skills to decide who plays each part within the fantasy. They also need to plan how the game will develop and to display reasoning when some of the children want to take it in a different direction. During fantasy play, children develop the essential ability to think before they act.

The developmental psychologist and children's play expert, Sara Smilansky, discovered that children who lacked the skills necessary for fantasy play also struggled in most areas of classroom learning. She found that high quality play could be taught by children to other children and appeared to be the "necessary precursor for every other kind of learning in a classroom".

There is a prevalent fashion for sitting children down and educating them before they are old enough for school. Smilansky's work shows that this will be counter-productive. The more time children spend playing, the better equipped they will become for classroom learning when they are older. I believe it is important for adults to be aware of this essential part of child development.

Social Play

Perhaps the greatest skill anyone can have in life is the ability to get on with other people. It is essential for work, friendships, deep relationships and happiness. It has always been an essential part of our evolution because our hunter-gatherer ancestors had to get along with each other so they could work together in the safety of groups. Play is a fundamental part of our evolution and it is superb at developing cooperation and empathy.

Imagine that Tom, Richard and Harry are playing together; however, if Tom won't let the other two play with his toys, then Richard and Harry are going to go and play by themselves. Tom does not enjoy playing by himself as much as playing with the other two, so he soon realises that he is going to have more fun if he lets Richard and Harry share his toys. As soon as Tom apologises and shares his toys, the other two forgive him because they all get to have a better play experience.

This process of cooperation works really well as long as the children who are unhappy with what is happening are free to leave the game. When adults step in and insist that Richard and Harry keep playing with Tom, saying things like, 'you shouldn't give up just because you are unhappy', or 'don't be mean by leaving Tom out', they are making not one, but two mistakes. First, Richard and Harry responded to their feelings about Tom's selfish behaviour in a natural way but they are now being told by adults that they were in the wrong. This makes Richard and Harry confused, angry and resentful of the adults who are supposed to be looking after them. It also teaches Tom that he can be as selfish as he likes and still get to play with all the other children. Play is extremely adept at developing a social and cooperative brain, but the whole process can be undermined by adult intervention.

If you are thinking that the adults would have explained to Tom that he ought to be a good boy and share his toys, and in doing so, Richard and Harry would then play with him, you are forgetting that a child's brain is not an adult brain in miniature. When information about how to behave is taught to children by adults, it enters the brain through the ears and is stored among the second level and third level processes, without involving the creation of brain pathways between the information and the primary instincts. The idea has been taught but it has not been experienced. When a child learns how to relate to other people via their instinctive play, the experience creates a link, a brain pathway, between the basic instincts and the appropriate behaviour. This is really important for two reasons: when play teaches a child to be sociable, the brain becomes wired-up to be sociable: however, when an adult teaches a child to be sociable, it is a piece of information stored in their memory, which may or may not modify a child's response to their emotions. If a child never forms the appropriate links between their basic, primal emotions and sociable behaviour, it can lead to huge problems later in life. When such a child becomes an adult, they may have difficulty forming happy relationships because they struggle to appreciate someone else's point of view.

No play

What happens to children if they have a childhood devoid of play? For obvious ethical reasons, we cannot conduct an experiment on children to find out, but Jaak Panksepp has done this work on rodents. He had a group of young rats which were all treated the same way, except some were allowed to play normally, whereas the others were never allowed to play. When they became adults, the play-deprived rats were extremely aggressive and anti-social. Rats are normally sociable creatures but these rats had no cooperative behaviour whatsoever. Their lack of play had prevented the normal development of relationship skills. The areas of the brain involved in play and social development are the oldest parts of the brain (in terms of evolution) and those structures are remarkably similar in humans and rats. It is, therefore, quite possible that children who are deprived of play will also grow up to be aggressive and anti-social. The length of time that children in the developed world spend on free play has been in steady decline for decades.

Dr Stuart Brown is the founder of the American National Institute for Play. He is a psychiatrist who has devoted his life to studying and promoting play because of his experiences when analysing the minds of murderers and other extremely violent men. He claims that the most violent people he has examined invariably had a childhood lacking in opportunities for free and natural play.[3] This lack of play gave them no consideration for other people and no proper control over their own emotional outbursts. His interest in this field began when he was one of the team analysing the mind of Charles Whitman. Whitman was a seemingly normal, 25-year-old, engineering student who, one afternoon in 1966, killed his wife and mother and then shot 58 other people, killing 17 of them, at the University of Texas. Dr Brown discovered that Whitman had a domineering and abusive father who would not let his young son go out to play nor allow friends to come home to play, with tragic consequences in later years.

However, Dr Brown has also observed a strong correlation between success in life and playful activity. Although the instinct to play is stronger in childhood, we all have the ability to be playful throughout our lives. He suggests that the happiest and most successful people we know are probably also the most playful. In an interview about play he said:

"An adult who has lost his playfulness becomes stereotyped, inflexible, humourless, lives without irony, loses the capacity for optimism, and generally is quicker to react to stress with violence or depression than the adult whose playfulness persists. In a world of major continuous change, playful humans who can roll with the punches and innovate through their play-inspired imaginations will survive better. Our playful natures have arrived at this moment in time through the trial and error of millions of years of evolution, and we need to honour our design to play."

Who stole our play?

The importance of play cannot be over-emphasised. For thousands of years our children have played, learned and developed with minimum interference from adults until the last few decades, during which society's attitudes to play and child development have changed. The time, space and opportunity for children to engage in spontaneous play have all drastically diminished in recent years. A study by Play England, an agency dedicated to encouraging play provision, showed that while 71% of parents had played outside their homes when young, only 21% of their own children were allowed that independence.[4] The distance children are allowed to roam from their homes has fallen from several miles to about a hundred metres. Many children living in cities never experience the natural world of woodland and green spaces and they rarely play out in the street with their neighbours. The reduction in opportunities for play has been so severe that experts have coined the phrase, 'play deprivation'. They fear that whole generations of children will grow up 'play deprived' and will suffer from an array of physical, psychological and social problems because of it.

Peter Gray is an American Professor of Psychology at Boston College who points out there has been a significant increase in anxiety and depression in young people during the last fifty to sixty years. In *The Decline of Play and the Rise of Psychopathology in Children and Adolescents* he cites studies which show that five to eight times more children and college students have clinical depression or anxiety than they did 50 years ago. Between 1950 and 2005 suicide rates quadrupled for children under 15 and doubled for young people aged between 15 and 25. Gray believes that the loss of unstructured, free play for play's sake is at the core of this alarming change and that as a society, we should reassess the role of free play and the factors which seem to have all but eliminated it from our children's lives.

What has caused this? Who are the big, bad bogeymen stealing play away from our children? Who are the nastiest trolls underneath the bridge of playfulness? There is a long list of villains in this tragic tale.

Fear is at the root of most of the changes which now prevent children from enjoying the experience of play, which was once a commonplace activity. That fear, of course, comes from the adults, not the children. Some of these new fears have a reasonable basis, but most do not. It is undoubtedly true that the number of vehicles on our roads has increased greatly in the last twenty years and in many places, where children used to play out in the street, it is now too busy with traffic to do so safely. On busy streets it is reasonable for parents to be worried about the safety of their children, although in many residential streets there are now speed bumps and other traffic calming measures to reduce the risk of collisions.

There is also the fear of 'stranger danger': the fear that your child may be abducted when out of your sight. This would, undoubtedly, be a terrible experience but it is extremely rare. We are all very aware of it because of the enormous amount of publicity when it does happen and, consequently, the fear it generates is completely out of proportion to the likelihood of it happening. More than half of all child abductions are committed by parents, other relatives or acquaintances, which means that, statistically speaking, your child is safer with a complete stranger than someone they know. Barry Glassner, a sociology professor in California and a fellow of Oxford University, wrote about missing children in his book *The Culture of Fear*:

"In national surveys conducted in recent years three out of four parents say they fear that their child will be kidnapped by a stranger. They harbour this anxiety, no doubt, because they keep hearing frightening statistics and stories about perverts snatching children off the street. What the public does not hear often or clearly enough is that the majority of missing children are runaways fleeing from physically or emotionally abusive parents."

Child abductions are an awful reality, but the risk should be kept in perspective. In his book, *Protecting the Gift*, child-safety expert Gavin De Becker pointed out that compared to being kidnapped by a stranger, "a child is vastly more likely to have a heart attack, and child heart attacks are so rare that most parents, quite correctly, never even consider the risk." The bogeyman in this instance is the media; they fuel your fears with long and detailed accounts of every aspect of the tragic action and prick your emotions with smiling pictures of the unfortunate child. There is a lack of balance here because a report saying, "millions and millions of children were not abducted again today" fails to be newsworthy.

Screens instead of play

Have you ever heard anyone complain that they bought an expensive toy but their child spent more time playing with the box it came in? The problem with some expensive toys is that the toy does the playing and the child is only superficially involved. A cardboard box, however, could be a car, a bus, a boat, a train, a space ship, a submarine, a cupboard, a table, a house, a cave or anything else that imagination will allow. A lot of toys nowadays are electronic, screen-based games and while there is nothing wrong with playing them, the length of time spent on them, or in front of a television screen, can be a huge problem.

A report by the Chief Medical Officer in 2013 showed that children who spend more time watching screens tend to have higher levels of emotional stress, anxiety and depression.[5] The report says:

"Long-term research suggests TV viewing at younger ages (one to three years old) predicts later attention and hyperactivity difficulties among seven-year-olds. Increased screen time and exposure to media (such as bedroom TVs) is consistently associated with reduced feelings of social acceptance, and increased feelings of loneliness, behaviour problems and aggression. Increased TV viewing is associated with lower self-worth and self-esteem and lower levels of self-reported happiness. The odds on children being worry-free were highest in those who watched less than an hour of TV on weekdays. Parents were also more likely to regard their child as unhappy if they watched a very large amount of TV. Specific types of internet activity (social networking sites, multi-player online games) have been associated with lower levels of wellbeing among children."

The report does not say why this happens, but several research studies suggest the reason is likely to be the more time a child spends in front of a TV or computer screen, the less time they have to engage in normal, active, healthy play. However, the report does go on to discuss physical activity:

"Physical activity is associated with improved concentration levels, more positive social behaviour, such as being kind to class mates and attempting to resolve disputes, and children feeling liked by peers and that they have enough friends. Physical activity is also associated with lower levels of anxiety and depression, with children being happier with their appearance, and reporting higher levels of self-esteem, happiness and satisfaction with their lives. Enjoying physical activity is also associated with happiness and lower levels of worry."

Why do so many children sit in front of a screen when it makes them stressed and unhappy? I think it is a combination of several factors. Companies make a lot of money from advertising their latest computer games but make nothing from promoting the benefits of playing in the park. The marketing people of electronic entertainment companies are working hard to promote their products, but when they are overused, they deprive children of the time for normal, outdoor play. Their financial success has been boosted considerably by the culture of fear and aversion to risk, which has escalated and spiralled out of control in recent years. Health and safety assessments began, many years ago, as sensible procedures to minimise risk in dangerous situations but they have expanded and extended their influence into every aspect of life, even where there is no realistic danger whatsoever. The agencies that oversee this juggernaut of interference and regulation are especially keen on child safety. You will hear their representatives say such things as, "We all have a duty to keep children safe," or "Child safety is paramount."

Whereas these statements sound earnest and profound, they are actually causing more harm than good. They imply that children must be protected from every possible danger, which is both impossible and undesirable. If you keep children indoors to protect them from meeting a paedophile, which has a risk of about 1 in 5 million, you expose them to the risk of developing obesity and other life-shortening diseases, which for sedentary children has a risk of about 1 in 3. Of course, if their time indoors is spent on social media websites, they have also increased their risk of exposure to paedophiles in a more insidious way. When anyone talks about keeping children safe, you need to ask, safe from what?

Government safety overkill

Professor Tanya Byron is a clinical psychologist and author of several books on children's mental health. She believes that children are being "raised in captivity" because of the "insane" levels of risk aversion. Back in 2009 she said, "Very rarely are children seen on the streets, playing outside, taking themselves to school because we live in such a risk averse and paranoid culture around child safety." She wrote a report for the Government on children's use of websites and video games. In it, she warned that far too many children were kept indoors because of parental fears about safety, but were then allowed free access to the internet where they were exposed to cyber-bullying and sexual predators.

In his book, *No Fear: Growing up in a risk averse society,* Tim Hill argues that childhood is "being undermined by the growth of risk aversion and its intrusion into every aspect of children's lives. This restricts children's play, limits their freedom of movement, corrodes their relationships with adults and constrains their exploration of physical, social and virtual worlds".

He discusses the Government's contribution to this awful mess and cites *The Safeguarding Vulnerable Groups Act* 2006 as a major step towards more risk aversion (and therefore worse outcomes for children). The idea was to make sure that people who worked with children, or vulnerable adults, had no previous record of inappropriate behaviour. This sounds like a good idea, but as Tim Hill points out: 'The Act places around nine million adults technically under suspicion of abuse: a third of the adult working population.' The Act, for the first time, extends mandatory vetting to include over two million volunteers and workers involved in sport and leisure activities, and over 200,000 school governors.

Governments of every type are very keen on producing new laws, but they all seem to be incapable of grasping the Law of Unintended Consequences. *The Safeguarding Vulnerable Groups*

Act was supposed to keep children safe from people who want to do them harm. What it has actually done is to assume that millions of adults, who volunteer to help with a huge range of children's activities, are potentially unsuitable or even dangerous, unless they can prove otherwise by paying about £60 for a Disclosure and Barring Service check (DBS, formerly known as CRB.) It has created an atmosphere of fear and mistrust between children and adults. As a result, large numbers of volunteers are giving up because of the insinuation, the cost and the danger that an innocent remark, or the slightest physical contact with a child, will result in an accusation of abuse, which will destroy not only their reputations but also their careers and perhaps even their lives. This law has greatly increased the aversion to risk in children's lives, which is one of the main destroyers of free play. Tim Hill concludes:

"Underpinning and connecting all these harmful tendencies is an assumption of children's vulnerability (or in the case of antisocial behaviour, their villainy) combined with failure to prioritise ways of fostering their resilience and sense of responsibility."

We have already looked at the evidence which illustrates that instinctive play is the best way to foster children's resilience and responsibility, but as a society we seem to be doing our utmost to prevent the proper development of young people. Our paranoia about safety, and fear of risk, has become so widespread and intense that it has spawned a culture of blame and litigious victimhood. While I agree that people who have been damaged by someone else's negligence should be able to seek compensation, I am horrified by the attitude that every accident must be someone's fault. If you put the words 'accident claim school' into an internet search engine, you get pages of law firms specialising in accident compensation. My dictionary defines 'accident' as 'an event that happens by chance without apparent or deliberate cause'. How can you sue someone for an accident? According to reports in the press, on average, education authorities in England settle two compensation claims of £7,500 each, every school day of the year.

A typical example of this occurred in 2013 and involved a six year old girl who fell over in the school playground after being bumped by another child who was playing tag. The girl cut her head on a wooden planter, which had passed health and safety checks, and her mother sued for compensation via her solicitor. The City Council decided to settle out of court and the girl received £1,100. However, the council had to pay the mother's legal costs of £13,000 as well as their own legal costs of £20,000. They decided to settle because they could not afford the legal costs if they had lost the case. The girl got £1,100 but the solicitors, between them, got £33,000. You and I paid out that money for a typical childhood accident. The judge involved in the case described it as "a complete waste of tax payers' money".

Compensation claims for childhood accidents cost the tax payer an enormous amount of money. As you can see from the example above, sometimes the lawyers get 30 times as much money as the girl who had the accident. Worse still, this culture of blame actively encourages the attitude that every mishap in life is someone else's fault and thereby diminishes the importance of personal responsibility. I regard personal responsibility as the corner-stone of a successful society. This compensation culture denies children the opportunity to learn from their own mistakes. Lastly, and by far the worst, is the damage this attitude is doing to children's play. Schools, education authorities and voluntary organisations are now terrified of being sued and their response is to cut back on every situation where children might fall over and graze their knees.

All of these health and safety initiatives begin with the best of intentions but they all snowball out of control. They so often make us neither healthy nor safe. The aversion to risk and the fear of litigation are making children far more sedentary and, indisputably, that makes them less healthy. Jaak Panksepp, Stuart Brown and other researchers have shown that children who are denied the opportunity for normal, instinctive, physically active play, grow up far more likely to be anti-social, violent and aggressive.

What can we do about this? We must do something. If you are in a dilemma and worrying about your children's safety, whilst also worrying about their lack of play and their sedentary life, there will no doubt be plenty of other parents nearby who feel the same. In some places, parents have been able to get together with others from their local school or neighbourhood and arrange for a large group of children to go off and play together at prearranged times. On other occasions, two or three parents from the group take children off into the woods to help them build dens, or whatever else they want to do.

If you cannot send your children out to play alone and you cannot find other people to form a play group, I recommend you send your children somewhere run by trained playworkers. Playwork is not childcare; it is a recognised qualification with a degree course in some British Universities. Playworkers provide places, facilities and equipment for play; they encourage play but they never direct it because they recognise that play is the child's business. One of their major principles states:

"Play is a process that is freely chosen, personally directed and intrinsically motivated. That is, children and young people determine and control the content and intent of their play, by following their own instincts, ideas and interests, in their own way for their own reasons". It is good news for children that we have playworkers, but a tragic indictment of society that we need them.

Summary
- Children's play is an instinctive and crucial activity in the development of a young brain.
- True play is directed by the children involved and any of them must be free to leave if they wish to.
- Play takes many forms and produces many benefits including empathy, creativity, courage, strength, balance and sociability.
- Children are engaging in real, outdoor play less and less with potentially dire consequences on their physical and mental well-being.

- The culture of absolute safety in children's activities is futile and counterproductive.

Chapter 16

HAPPINESS

Happiness is a sense of contentment, well-being and comfort. When I talk about happiness, I am not talking about the sense of euphoria you feel when something wonderful happens. Nor am I talking about the despair you feel when something goes horribly wrong. The extreme emotional reactions caused by major events in our lives are things we all have to deal with and I cannot help you with your personal twists of fate. However, there are things we can all do to improve the baseline level of our daily happiness and contentment. We are all in need of more happiness.

According to the Nuffield Trust:

'The proportion of children and young people saying they have a mental health condition has grown six fold in England over two decades and has increased significantly across the whole of Britain in recent years. The age group with the biggest increases were people aged 16-24, with young people in England almost 10 times more likely to report a long-standing mental health condition in 2014 than in 1995.'

Medicines prescribed for anxiety, depression, obsessive-compulsive disorder and panic attacks rose from 31 million in 2006 to 65 million in 2016: a rise of 108%. The numbers of people self-harming, committing suicide and being detained under the Mental Health Act are all rising. A tragic lack of happiness is accelerating in our society and we must do something about it. The government and their advisers say we need more mental health services, more psychologists and psychiatrists and more money to pay for them all. These are all important but, as with physical health, they are not asking the right question: "Why are so many people suffering from mental illness?'

Prevention of mental decline is a better approach than trying to cure a well-established problem. Prevention is achieved by understanding what happiness is and how to maintain it. The first thing to realise is that pleasure and happiness are not the same thing. The best explanation I have found to describe the difference between these two sensations is given by Dr Robert Lustig in his book, *The Hacking of the American Mind:*

- *Pleasure is short-lived; happiness is long-lived.*
- *Pleasure is visceral; happiness is ethereal.*
- *Pleasure is taking; happiness is giving.*
- *Pleasure can be achieved with substances; happiness cannot be achieved with substances.*
- *Pleasure is experienced alone; happiness is experienced in social groups.*
- *The extremes of pleasure all lead to addiction, whether they be substances or behaviours. There is no such thing as being addicted to too much happiness.*
- *Pleasure is tied to the brain chemical dopamine and happiness is tied to the brain chemical serotonin.*

Doing things which give us pleasure is an important part of a happy life as long as we do not become obsessed with the feelings of pleasure. Dopamine is a molecule released in the brain when we experience something pleasurable. Dopamine excites the nerve receptors it interacts with and this reaction gives rise to the feeling of pleasure. However, when those receptors are overstimulated for an extended period of time, they protect themselves by reducing their sensitivity. This process is known as down-regulation, or tolerance, and when it begins we need a bigger dose of dopamine to get the same level of pleasure. A bigger dose, however, creates more down-regulation and a need for more stimulation. Eventually, we can become addicted to the source of our original pleasure although it gives us little of the enjoyment we seek. Too much of a particular substance, or activity, leads to unwanted side-effects, guilt and a decline in many aspects of life.

Serotonin is also a nerve-stimulating molecule in the brain but it does not over-excite its nerve cell receptors and does not lead to addiction. It gives us a feeling of happiness and contentment. Dopamine makes us think, 'I like this and I want more', while serotonin makes us think, 'I like this but I do not need or want more'. The awful irony is that dopamine can make us less sensitive to serotonin. This means that the more we become addicted to pleasure, the less able we are to enjoy happiness.

A great deal of our modern world is full of situations that stimulate dopamine and reduce serotonin. Young people are suffering the most from mental disorders, partly because they are exposed to dopamine stimulators more than older people. Social media is like a dopamine factory because it encourages everyone to connect with other people, so they will connect with you. Thinking, for a fleeting moment, that someone else likes you, likes your picture, what you said or the colour of your shirt produces a quick burst of pleasure: a quick burst of dopamine. There is nothing satisfying in these feelings, so we often seek more of them in the hope of feeling better.

When we have a thousand friends on Facebook, we imagine that we must be very popular but these are not real friends. Real friends would stop what they are doing and come to help us if we were truly in need of help. How many Facebook 'friends' would do that? How much time do we have for our real friends when we are swapping 'likes' with a thousand 'virtual friends'?

We are bombarded with advertising for all sorts of things we do not need. The models in these adverts always appear to be more beautiful, successful and wealthy than we are. The advertisers think you will buy their products because you want to be like the people in the advert. A lot of people do so, but when the dopamine hit at the time of purchase wears off, we realise that our expensive new gadget does not make us beautiful, successful nor wealthy. Instead, it leaves us feeling acutely aware of our own perceived inadequacies and limitations. This feeling reduces our serotonin levels and our baseline happiness. In the past people became rich or famous because of what they had done and achieved. Nowadays some people achieve celebrity status because of how they look and how flagrantly they are prepared to show it off. We can feel respect for someone's hard work and dedication but we are more likely to feel jealousy when someone earns excessive amounts of money for apparently little effort.

We would expect older people to suffer from more mental health problems than young people because of the natural decline that happens with ageing. While the elderly certainly have an increased incidence of dementia and Alzheimer's disease, the latest research shows that there is a peak of mental ill-health among people in their twenties, which declines steadily as we get older. Happy people care more about how good their friends are, not how many friends they appear to have.

Robert Lustig, who I mentioned earlier, thinks that the global corporations which dominate the retail world know exactly what they are doing. He believes they are creating products designed specifically to stimulate dopamine in our brains so we will keep coming back to spend more and more of our money on more and more of their products. Many young people feel they absolutely have to have the latest smart phone, for example. The tragedy is that the things they think they want are contributing to their declining mental health and denying them the thing they need most, which is happiness.

Shortened attention span is another increasing problem and nothing diminishes attention span like a flashing screen, a beeping noise or a photo that disappears in a few seconds. Research has shown that simply having a phone on your desk whilst working, significantly diminishes concentration on the task at hand. Even when the phone is switched off, its presence in your peripheral vision is distracting because part of your brain wants to see what your favourite celebrity had for breakfast, or whatever it is that your particular dopamine hit is triggered by.

How to increase our happiness
There are various ways to diminish dopamine and increase serotonin and thereby increase happiness. These methods are precisely what people used to do before the advertising world hijacked our brains. As I mentioned in Chapter 3, this is exactly how indigenous tribes live, and it is almost impossible to find mental illness among those egalitarian societies.

1. Relate to people.

Spend more time talking, and listening, to real friends, family and colleagues. Look them in the eye as you concentrate on the dialogue between you. This builds empathy on both sides and empathy increases self-esteem, which is a serotonin experience. What we should not do, is to go out with a group of friends and all sit around a table looking at our mobile phones. That is a dopamine experience.

2. Give freely.

The act of helping people out of kindness, without seeking something in return, is a noble, serotonin-boosting thing to do. When people realise you have helped them for no reward, they are much more likely to do the same for you and everybody benefits. But if you trick and cheat your way through life, you won't experience happiness and when you are in need of help, there is going to be nobody there to provide it.

3. Develop a sense of community.

We evolved in small groups because our distant ancestors realised we were all better off if we helped each other. The immediate area around our home has a big impact on our lives and we should make the most of it. Do you know your neighbours? Do you talk to them? Do you and they do anything to keep your street clean and tidy? Do you feel part of a community?

4. Give life purpose and meaning.

In the words of the famous Swiss psychoanalyst, Carl Jung, "The least of things with a meaning is worth more in life than the greatest of things without it." To enjoy true happiness and contentment we need a sense of purpose. Each of us must decide for ourselves what brings meaning to our lives; it can range from securing world peace to making sure you walk the dog every day. Jung is saying that it does not matter what your purpose is, as long as you have one, or even more than one.

5. Take regular exercise.

As I said in Chapter 12, regular physical activity reduces stress and boosts beneficial brain chemicals, especially when it is done outside in green spaces. Exercise is surprisingly good at boosting our mood and our sense of physical well-being. Or perhaps it isn't surprising, when we remember how important it was for our ancestors to walk and run every day to catch all the meat they used to eat.

6. Embrace playfulness.

Our instinct for play may diminish when we reach adulthood but it does not leave us altogether. The word is etched into our language: we play golf, cards and football. We go to the theatre to watch a play; comedy is a play on words. My thesaurus links play with frolic, frisk, gambol, romp, cavort and caper. They all sound like fun things to do and I wonder how long it is since most of us did any of them? A playful frame of mind is very resistant to depression.

7. Sleep.

None of us can function properly without adequate sleep. A sleep deficiency disrupts our hormones making us more irritable and stressed. It is vitally important for children, throughout their childhood, to have a dark, quiet bedroom where they can obtain all the sleep they need.

Stress

Prolonged periods of excessive stress can lead to physical and mental ill-health brought on by the over-production of the hormone cortisol. These problems can include the following:

- Decreased immunity leading to more frequent colds and infections.
- Chronic fatigue and lower energy levels.
- Disrupted sleep patterns and increased insomnia.
- Reduced libido. Some studies have found that higher levels of stress are associated with less sexual desire, arousal and satisfaction. It can also cause irregular periods in women.
- Increased frequency of headaches.
- Increased blood sugar levels, which cause increased insulin production. As we know, this leads to weight gain, high blood pressure, and eventually, type 2 diabetes.
- Loss of appetite or a ravenous hunger with binge-eating.

- Increased skin problems. The stress hormone, cortisol, can induce acne, slow-healing wounds, bruising and stretch marks on the stomach, hips and thighs.
- Studies have shown a link between stress and digestive disorders ranging from constipation and diarrhoea, to irritable bowel syndrome.
- Stress also makes us more emotional and is associated with increased episodes of depression.

Mild, short-term stress is a normal part of life and the hormonal changes that occur are designed to help us to cope with it. Long-term, severe stress is far from normal and we are not well equipped to deal with it. An internet search will reveal a wide range of ideas for reducing stress. However, most of them advise things like 'take a warm bath, surrounded by soothing music and scented candles'. I expect this works well if you have had a tough day at work but I do not think it is going to take away your stress if you have lost your job and do not know how to pay your mortgage.

Dealing with stress depends on the level of stress we may be facing. Big problems in our lives need to be dealt with. We need to be brave and make whatever changes are required to eliminate major stress from our daily lives. We need to recognise the problem, talk about the problem and try to alter it. For many people, however, stress comes simply from being too busy and trying to juggle too many responsibilities. In this situation, we tend to think we do not have the time for all the things that reduce stress, like outdoor exercise, yoga, meditation and eating a meal together. The reality is that making time for these activities does reduce stress, which enables us to deal with our difficulties much more efficiently.

Food for the brain
It is widely accepted that a poor diet contributes to a decline in physical health so it is logical to assume that a bad diet would also influence mental health. There are two modern trends in food consumption that have a negative impact on our brains.

We have already looked at the many physical problems of eating too much sugar and refined carbohydrate. However, it is worth remembering that a spike in blood sugar is followed by a spike in insulin, which brings the glucose level back down. The combination of falling sugar levels and increased insulin trigger the production of stress hormones, which increase anxiety. Repeated snacking on sugary food creates a rollercoaster of mood swings, which are the antithesis of the calmness and serenity experienced during true happiness. A 1995 study, published in the *Journal of Pediatrics* by Dr W. Tamborlane, showed that teenage boys who drank sugar-sweetened drinks had adrenaline levels five times higher than boys consuming no sugar, four hours after the test began. Adrenaline is one of the 'flight or fight' hormones which make us agitated and aggressive.

We know that too much carbohydrate leads to insulin resistance, which in turn leads to type 2 diabetes and all the physical problems associated with that disease. However, it is becoming apparent that high levels of blood sugar and insulin are also causing defects in normal brain function. People with bipolar disorder are 300% more likely to have diabetes than people without those problems.[1]   This information comes from an observational study and therefore cannot prove that bipolar is caused by high blood sugar but on the Grade system, as mentioned previously, this 300% relates to a hazard ratio of 3. This is much more significant than the 1.18 ratio used by The World Health Organisation, and others, to suggest that red meat is a likely cause of colon cancer. The WHO report led to a deluge of media coverage asking us all to cut back on meat. Why is there no campaign against excess carbohydrate to prevent bipolar disorder when the risk is far greater? Could it be that the processed food industry makes a huge amount of money out of sugar and refined carbohydrates and the pharmaceutical industry makes a huge amount of money out of drugs for mental disorders? Neither of these financial superpowers want you to eat real food from your local farmer because they cannot make any profit out of that.

Schizophrenia is regarded as the close cousin of bipolar disorder. It is an awful and long-lasting psychotic condition in which people are unable to distinguish between their own thoughts and reality. Dr Chris Palmer is a psychiatrist from Harvard

Medical School. He has published a paper[2] about two schizophrenic patients, who had both taken a large selection of powerful drugs and undergone electroconvulsive therapy over many years. Their conditions remained severe. They were both overweight and, independently, decided to use a ketogenic diet to shed their excess pounds. Within weeks they each showed huge improvement in their symptoms and, as a bonus, they also lost weight. Dr Palmer stated that the improvement in their mental health on the ketogenic diet was far greater than any drug or therapy had been able to achieve.

In Chapter 6, we learnt that Alzheimer's disease is now being referred to by some researchers as type 3 diabetes because 80% of people with Alzheimer's disease display insulin resistance. All these mental disorders are linked to high levels of blood sugar caused by a diet of too many carbohydrates. These mental health disorders exist on a sliding scale; just because you don't have a diagnosis of mental ill health, does not mean that your brain chemistry is not compromised by too much sugar and insulin. People who change from the officially recommended high-carbohydrate diet to a low-carbohydrate, high-fat diet frequently enthuse about their new sense of mental clarity.

The other trend that has great potential to damage our brain function is veganism. I mentioned this in Chapter 10, but it is worth repeating. Two thirds of our brains are made of fat molecules and 20% of all that fat consists of an omega 3 fatty acid known as DHA. DHA is essential for a multitude of processes in the brain and some neurologists suggest that conscious thought is impossible without it. There is no DHA in plant foods; we can only obtain it from animal sources. (It is possible to convert a plant based omega 3 known as ALA into DHA but the process is very inefficient and vegans invariably display much lower levels than omnivores.)

Vitamin B12 is also essential for healthy brain function. A published case study from Scandinavia[3] describes a woman in her 50s with anxiety, movement abnormalities, constipation, lethargy, perceptual disturbances and catatonia. Despite receiving the full range of standard treatments in hospital, she remained suicidal, depressed and lethargic. Eventually, she was given vitamin B12 injections and all her symptoms disappeared and she remains symptom free years afterwards. Another case report [4] describes a woman in her 60s:

'She seemed sad and older than her real age. Facial expression and spontaneous movements were reduced, her speech and movements were very slow. She had depressed mood, guilt complex, incurability and devaluation impressions. She had Capgras' syndrome and delusion of persecution.' (People with Capgras' syndrome believe a close relative or friend has been replaced with an imposter.) All her symptoms were resolved nine days after starting a course of vitamin B12 injections and iron replacement.

Vitamin B12 is completely absent from a vegan's diet unless they take supplements or eat certain fermented foods or algae. It is found abundantly in animal-based foods and even people who are persuaded to reduce their meat consumption and increase the plants in their diet, run the risk of sub-optimal levels of B12 and DHA. An entirely plant-based diet cannot supply the essential ingredients for a happy brain.

Young people are suffering unprecedented levels of mental ill-health. There are, of course, many complex reasons for it, but the under-30s are the demographic group most likely to be vegan or vegetarian and least likely to think of food in terms of its nutrient content. We all need to be aware of how important good food is for mental health and to teach our children this vital information.

Eating enough protein is also important for a happy brain. There are nine essential amino acids that we all have to eat to make the proteins we need. Tryptophan is one of these amino acids and a good supply is necessary for the brain to able to create the 'happiness molecule': serotonin. A publication entitled *The Effects of Dietary Tryptophan on Affective Disorders*, by Glenda Lindseth, covers most of the research done on this topic. Many of the quoted studies have shown that the depletion of tryptophan levels is closely linked to increased rates of depression and anxiety. The reverse is also true. A study was conducted as a two-phase trial involving 24 participants with mania, some of whom consumed large doses of tryptophan over a two week period. Using standard tests, the authors of the study found that the severity of mania symptoms was significantly reduced in the group taking tryptophan. Many of the researchers found that tryptophan was most useful for people who had already suffered from depression or anxiety and were, therefore, most likely to be depleted in serotonin. However, the authors of this research demonstrated that healthy individuals showed significantly improved mood when they consumed high levels of tryptophan compared to consuming low levels. An important proviso is that these people were also supplied with a good source of vitamin B6, which is essential in the production of neuro-transmitters, like serotonin. Vitamin B6 is found in a wide range of unprocessed foods including poultry, eggs, liver and fish.

This all demonstrates that a healthy brain is just as dependent on the correct diet as is a healthy body. The fatty acid DHA, vitamin B12 and tryptophan are all vital ingredients for the experience of happiness. They can all be obtained from eating unprocessed animal foods like eggs, fish, meat or poultry. To consume enough DHA, we need to eat the fat that naturally comes with the protein, just like our distant ancestors did. Never forget that the concept of 'lean meat' was a political compromise invented by American Senators. It has no foundation in nutritional science.

Summary.
- Pleasure is not the same thing as happiness.
- Mental health problems are increasing in a world dominated by addictive technology.
- Giving freely to other people, a sense of community, a sense of purpose, regular exercise, playfulness and sleep all tend to boost our happiness.
- Too much stress inhibits happiness.
- A diet high in animal fat and protein is essential for optimum brain function.

Chapter 17

WHAT TO EAT

Throughout this book, I have tried to demonstrate that most of the things we are told about how to be healthy are wrong. This is especially true about our food. It is, therefore, important for me to list the things we should be eating. The simple answer is real food: unprocessed, home cooked food that comes from a farm or a fisherman and not a factory. Recent studies have shown that 51% of the food bought in the UK is ultra-processed, and the UK is the fattest, most unhealthy country in Europe. Before we look at what we should eat, let us look at what we should not eat.

The word 'processed', when applied to food, can cover a wide range of procedures. Packaged vegetables that have been cleaned and chopped ready for cooking could be called processed, but in reality they have simply been prepared for the sake of convenience. We should all avoid ultra-processed food that has undergone considerable alteration from its natural form. This kind of food will contain substances with no nutritional value which are added to increase shelf-life, texture, colour and flavour. Some of the added ingredients are detrimental to health. Bread, for instance, used to be made from wheat flour, water, salt and yeast. Now it also contains soya flour, rapeseed oil and palm oil. Soya flour contains phytoestrogens that disrupt our hormones and rapeseed oil contributes to an excess of omega 6 fatty acids which increase inflammation in our bodies.

Cakes and biscuits have no part in a healthy diet. A typical supermarket chocolate cake has the following ingredients: sugar, wheat flour, dark brown sugar, rapeseed oil, butter, pasteurised egg, fat-reduced cocoa powder, water, glucose syrup, humectant (glycerol), dark chocolate, pasteurised egg white, cornflour, whole milk, golden syrup, milk chocolate, invert sugar syrup, raising agents (disodium diphosphate, potassium bicarbonate), cocoa mass, emulsifiers (mono- and di-glycerides of fatty acids), salt, preservative (potassium sorbate).

The first and most abundant ingredient is sugar followed by wheat flour which digests down to glucose. Dark brown sugar, glucose syrup, golden syrup and invert sugar syrup are just other names for sugar. A humectant is used in many processed foods to keep the food moist and extend shelf life. Emulsifiers are used to mix fat and water and produce a smooth texture. They can be found in everything from cosmetics and paint, to processed food. Recent research suggests that emulsifiers are causing considerable problems.

Our intestines are teeming with bacteria and most of them are entirely beneficial. The type of food we eat alters the balance between different strains of bacteria, causing significant effects on our health. We did not evolve to eat ultra-processed food and neither did our gut microbiome. Our intestinal wall is protected from all these bacteria by a mucosal layer. Emulsifiers don't just emulsify fat and water in food, they are quite happy to emulsify our mucosal layer as well. Damage to this layer allows gut bacteria to access the lining of the intestines, increasing the chance of inflammatory bowel diseases. Irritable bowel syndrome, Celiac and Crohn's disease have all increased dramatically during the last sixty years, in line with the increased intake of processed food containing too much sugar, inflammatory seed oils and emulsifiers. These three things are abundant in almost every single processed food and provide no health benefits whatsoever.

Highly processed food provides something else we have not evolved to deal with: an abnormal mix of fat and sugar. Naturally occurring foods rarely contain high levels of fat and carbohydrate together. We get fat and protein together in animal foods, and carbohydrate with some protein in plant foods but only in modern, processed foods do we get large amounts of fat and sugar. We evolved with a brain-based craving for sugary foods, which produce a dopamine response. This encouraged us to eat plenty of carbohydrate when it was available and store it as fat for times when food was scarce. We also have a liking for foods containing fat because that was the main source of energy throughout our evolution. A study, published in 2018 by Yale University, in *Cell Metabolism*, examined this process. Among their conclusions they said: "We theorize that the simultaneous activation of fat and carbohydrate signalling pathways launches an effect that human physiology has not evolved to handle. Consistent with this suggestion, rodents given access to fat alone or carbohydrate alone regulate their total daily calorie intake and body weight. But given unrestricted access to fat and carbohydrates, they quickly gain weight".

The conclusion is simple: modern ultra-processed foods like cakes, biscuits, doughnuts, chocolate bars and 'potato-based snacks' hijack our appetite control centre causing us to overeat. These fake foods are designed to make us eat too much and when we do so, we become fat and ill. If we want to be healthy, we have to stop eating ready-made, ultra-processed food. Ditching all this fake food will improve our health. It might also save us some time when we go shopping: in a typical supermarket, there are probably about 10 aisles that you will never need to walk down again because they do not contain any real food.

There is some confusion about processed meat. The World Health Organisation has declared that it causes colorectal cancer. I discussed the weak evidence for this claim in Chapter 10, demonstrating the evidence came from observational studies and is compounded by the fact that people who eat a lot of processed meat also tend to eat lots of other processed food. What I did not mention previously is the fact that the WHO has entered into formal, cooperative partnerships with the Seventh Day Adventist Church in various parts of the world. As we now know, that Church is the world's richest and most active voice for vegetarianism. Can we trust the WHO to be impartial about meat when they work with an organisation vehemently opposed to all meat products?

The term 'processed meat' covers a wide range of products from dry cured bacon and traditional salami to ultra-processed, factory produced hot dog sausages. The health worry comes from the addition of nitrates as preservatives. Laboratory tests have shown that nitrates, when heated, can react with amino acids to produce nitrosamines, which are thought to increase the chance of cancer. The problem is that nitrates occur naturally in a wide variety of vegetables. We are encouraged to eat beetroot, spinach and celery because they contain high levels of nitrates, which are converted to nitric oxide and, as we have seen, nitric oxide lowers blood pressure. It appears that official advice says that nitrates in vegetables are good but nitrates in meat are bad.

On October 1st 2019, the *Annals of Internal Medicine* published a report on the evidence behind the recommendation to limit the consumption of meat.[1] The study was conducted by 14 scientists from seven countries, who were all carefully vetted to exclude anyone with conflicts of interest. They said that the evidence against eating both fresh and processed meat was too weak and unreliable to be used in official dietary guidelines. Their conclusion stated: '*The panel suggests that adults continue current unprocessed red meat consumption and current processed meat consumption.*'

This study was widely reported in the media but frequently referred to as 'controversial'. We live in an era where the work of independent scientists, who insist on the highest standards of research, are regarded as controversial if their conclusions differ from the orthodoxy of the day.

It is hard to be definitive about processed meat and I think everybody has to make up their own mind. I absolutely recommend fresh meat and I have no fear of eating bacon or the type of salami you would find in a traditional Italian deli. However, I never eat anything as highly processed as a hot dog sausage.

The best way to reduce any risk of ill health from eating meat is to roast it, or fry it, in stable fats like lard, beef dripping, coconut oil or butter and avoid unstable poly-unsaturated seed oils, which we know can increase the risk of cancer. It might also be wise to avoid food that has been overcooked to the point of turning charred and black. However, the official advice to eat only lean meat is looking worse and worse. The fat of cattle and sheep contains fatty acids known as conjugated linoleic acids. These are a group of naturally occurring fat molecules which have been shown to hinder the development of cancerous cells. It appears that eating the fat that naturally comes with beef and lamb reduces the chance of developing cancer. This research was published in the British Journal of Nutrition by a group of French researchers under the title, *'Beef conjugated linoleic acid isomers reduce human cancer cell growth even when associated with other beef fatty acids'*.

What to eat?

For optimum health, we all need to eat a diet of unprocessed, whole food with low levels of carbohydrate and decent levels of natural fats and protein. We should eat when we are hungry and stop when we are full. If we eat meals with adequate fat and protein, and very little carbohydrate, we will feel satiated for long periods of time and have no need or desire for snacks in between. The idea of 'snacks to keep you going' between meals is a marketing trick by the fake food industry. If you feel hungry an hour after your last meal, it is a clear sign that your meal contained too much carbohydrate and you are experiencing the sugar-insulin rollercoaster. If we were to eat no carbohydrate at all, as some people do, our blood sugar would remain constant and optimal. It is possible to demonstrate this now by wearing a continuous blood glucose monitor. (There is a proviso: a sudden release of stress hormones can elevate blood sugar in preparation for a flight-or-fight response.) If we do not eat carbohydrate, the liver makes all the glucose we need via a process called glycogenesis.

How much carbohydrate is the right amount? The correct answer to that question is: it depends. The oft repeated mantra about eating everything in moderation is too simplistic. If you would not give a moderate amount of whisky to an alcoholic, you should not give a moderate amount of sugar to a diabetic. The amount of carbohydrate people can safely eat depends on how insulin sensitive or resistant they are. An endurance athlete with very high insulin sensitivity may be able to eat large amounts of carbohydrate without gaining any weight. (Sadly, I know of a few good distance runners and endurance athletes who continued to eat a high carbohydrate diet after their days of hard training had finished, and they are now type 2 diabetics.) Someone with severe insulin resistance has to restrict their carbohydrate intake considerably, and will need to limit their consumption to a maximum of 25 grams a day, which is the equivalent to one apple. People who are obese or already have diabetes fall into this category, and it is essential that they greatly restrict their carbohydrate intake to avoid amputations, blindness and an early death from heart disease, cancer or dementia.

People who are in between these two extremes of insulin resistance, but would like to lose weight, should reduce carbohydrate intake until their weight starts to fall naturally and then never go back above that level. Everybody should stop drinking sugar and eating refined, ultra-processed carbohydrates like sweets, cakes and biscuits for the sake of their long-term metabolic health. To lose weight, people with moderate insulin resistance also need to cut back on starchy foods like potatoes, rice, bread and pasta.

When we reduce carbohydrate intake, we have to increase the amount of fat we eat in order to maintain energy levels. The important thing to grasp here is that healthy fats are extremely good for our metabolic health and they are not to be feared. Some of the ways in which we can increase fat intake include:

- Swap skimmed or semi-skimmed milk for whole milk. Choose full fat cheese and natural yoghurt over reduced fat versions. Add sour cream to savoury stews or curries.

- Cook meat, fish, eggs and even vegetables with healthy fats like butter, lard, dripping, olive oil or coconut oil. Never cook with 'vegetable' oils.

- If you like to steam vegetables, add a knob of butter (and a little salt) to them once they are drained of water.

- Add high fat foods as a garnish on your meals. The Italians put parmesan cheese on top of many dishes. Try using other cheeses, diced bacon, chopped nuts, small pieces of avocado or olives.

- Eat more eggs. Eggs are one of the most nutrient dense foods we can ever eat. They are cheap and versatile. They contain vitamins A, E, D, K, B1, B6 and B12. They are rich in essential, omega 3 fatty acids like DHA. They contain protein as well as calcium, iron, zinc, phosphorus, copper, manganese and selenium. They are also one of the best sources of choline, which is essential for growth and development.

- Choose cuts of meat which are not too lean. Do not cut the fat off a piece of meat. Eating some of the fat and meat together improves the flavour and tenderness.

Some people, especially if they have metabolic syndrome, can benefit greatly from severe carbohydrate restriction. This type of low-carbohydrate, high-fat diet becomes a ketogenic diet when the body switches to using fat molecules, known as ketones, as its primary energy source. We have already seen that a ketogenic diet can be extraordinarily useful in some forms of epilepsy and the reversal of the symptoms of type 2 diabetes.

All types of animal foods are suitable for a low-carbohydrate diet. Beef, lamb, pork, fish, poultry, eggs, cheese, milk, cream and yoghurt are highly nutritious and have a very limited effect on insulin levels. Vegetables growing above the ground are generally low in carbohydrate and are suitable for people wanting to lose weight and improve their metabolic health. Typical choices would include: spinach, cabbage, broccoli, cauliflower, brussels sprouts, peppers, tomatoes, onions, mushrooms, asparagus, aubergines, courgettes, lettuce, leeks and avocado. Some vegetables, such as carrots, peas, butternut squash and sweet potatoes, have moderate carbohydrate levels and should only be eaten occasionally if you are trying to lose weight. Vegetables from under the ground, such as turnips, parsnips and potatoes, are mainly starch and will cause high blood sugar and insulin. They have little nutritional value and a lot of carbohydrate.

Fruits and vegetables are usually grouped together in nutritional advice, but their carbohydrate content can be vastly different. Modern varieties of most fruits are too high in sugar to be regarded as healthy options. Many people eat them because they are high in vitamin C, which is a useful anti-oxidant. However, molecules of glucose and vitamin C enter cells in the body via a shared transport system across the membrane. They compete with each other for access and, in the presence of high levels of glucose, very little vitamin C enters the cells to do its work.[2] The less carbohydrate we eat, the less vitamin C we need to eat. This is why people who only eat fresh meat and no plant foods do not get scurvy. Interestingly, carnivores who eat only tinned meat do get scurvy: freshness is important.

If you are worried about the cost of eating real food compared to processed food, it is worth remembering that we get what we pay for. Processed food is cheap because the ingredients are cheap. As supermarkets have come to dominate the sale of food, this has led to a price war as they attempt to gain market share. This process has drip-fed the idea that food is, and should be, cheap. In 1957, when the nation was considerably more healthy than it is now, households spent 33% of their disposable income on food. We now spend between 10% and 15%. Our attitude and priorities have changed, and our health has plunged in line with our spending on quality food.

Let me ask a hypothetical question. If your choice of food is based largely on cost, and you decide to eat processed food because it is cheaper than real food, you are more likely to become overweight, insulin resistant and, finally, diabetic. If you continue to eat badly as a diabetic, you may find yourself in need of an operation to amputate your foot or lower leg. Before you go into the operating theatre, how much would you be willing to pay for a medicine that could instantly reverse all the damage your diet has caused? I imagine most people would be willing to pay considerably more than they would have spent buying real food in the first place. In England and Wales, 6,000 people have a foot or leg amputated every year because of type 2 diabetes. This tragedy is completely avoidable with the correct diet.

Eating a healthy, nutritious, low-carbohydrate diet does not have to be any more expensive than an unhealthy, processed-food diet. You no longer need to buy breakfast cereals, cakes, biscuits, fizzy drinks, crisps, snacks and puddings. You do not need any of those things because you will spend less time each day feeling hungry. If you are lucky enough still to have a local butcher's shop, you can get plenty of advice from them on cheaper cuts of meat which are just as nutritious but less popular than steak. A local fishmonger can provide the same service.

If cooking real food from scratch is an uncommon event for your family, the benefits of a healthier diet will be immense. It will, however, take some effort to make the change. There are plenty of books and online courses to learn how to cook well. Producing home cooked meals is a source of great pride and satisfaction and, for some people, it can be one of life's important purposes. It does not have to be the responsibility of one person in a household. The more input that everyone has towards the production of tasty, healthy meals, which are enjoyed by the whole family, the more everyone appreciates the experience. When wholesome family meals become a regular, happy experience it is much more likely that the younger members of the family will continue to cook good food throughout their lives.

Children's food

On the subject of younger members of the family, why do we feed children so much sugar? One third of British children are overweight or obese when they leave Primary School and that problem is caused by what they eat. Children should eat the same healthy diet as adults eat, but they are relentlessly encouraged to eat snacks and sweets that have only calories and no nutritional value whatsoever. Some people might think they are giving their children a treat when they give them a fizzy drink and a bag of multi-coloured sweets. What they are actually giving them is tooth decay, weight gain and metabolic ill health.

The Government has realised that some children go to school without any breakfast and, therefore, have organised breakfast clubs, which provide a meal for these children at school before lessons begin. This sounds like a good idea but the devil is always in the details. A lot of schools rely on an outside organisation to provide the meals for these hungry children. A typical example of such an organisation might be feeding over 40,000 children each school day, and they proudly claim that their service leaves no child too hungry to learn. Unfortunately, they feed the children with food that does not help them to learn. Four items are typically provided: a bowl of breakfast cereal; a bowl of porridge; a bagel; and a glass of fruit juice. These organisations state that their meals are low in 'sugar, fat and salt'. However, the main ingredient in each of the items listed is carbohydrate, carbohydrate, carbohydrate and carbohydrate. As we know, starchy foods digest down to glucose, which means their healthy breakfasts are almost entirely sugar. Fat, from which our brains are made, is almost non-existent. Why do they not just give the children eggs every morning?

A child's health begins in the womb and a pregnant woman needs to eat a highly nutritious diet. I have already mentioned, in Chapter 10, that children born to vegan mothers can suffer from extreme neurological defects because their food lacks so many essential nutrients. However, you do not need to be vegan to have an inadequate diet. Recent research is suggesting that autism is linked to mineral and vitamin deficiencies in the mother during pregnancy.[3] A diet low in carbohydrate and high in healthy fats and protein made with fresh, unprocessed food is important for everybody and this approach is essential when you are growing a new person inside you.

Breastfeeding a baby for the first six months is vitally important, as long as it is possible. I am dumbfounded by people who object to mothers breastfeeding in public places; it is the most natural thing in the world. Creating barriers to it can have a negative impact on the number of mothers who do breastfeed. Weaning children onto real food is a process that global corporations see as an opportunity to make huge profits, but parents can easily make their own pureed food from fresh ingredients. The majority of websites giving advice on weaning suggest introducing a baby to solid food in the form of mashed fruit or potato, baby breakfast cereals and baby breadsticks. Most of the advice is for high carbohydrate, starchy food. Adults have no requirement for carbohydrate and neither do babies. Babies are born in a state of ketosis, meaning they are using ketones as their primary source of fuel when they arrive in the world. While starchy foods may be the best option to get a baby used to the texture of food, once they will take food from a spoon you can introduce them to a pureed, or mashed, version of the fatty meat and above ground vegetables you are eating by blending some of your own meal to a consistency your baby will eat. (Do so before adding salt because very young kidneys should not be exposed to too much salt.) It is both important, and easier in the long run, to start healthy eating habits from a young age.

The importance of animal foods for child development has been the subject of some important research.[4] In 2014 the *British Journal of Nutrition* published the results of a trial among Kenyan children. Nutritional deficiencies are all too common in rural Kenya, which is why this location was chosen. Twelve primary schools were involved and they were randomly allocated different diets, which they received over a two-year period. The groups ate a local plant-based stew with either added meat, added milk or nothing added at all. The researchers stated, "Children in the Meat group showed significantly greater improvements in test scores than those in all the other groups, and the Milk group showed significantly greater improvements in test scores than the Control group".

A study from the Brown School at Washington University in St. Louis, in 2017, found infants who were introduced to eggs from the age of 6 months, showed significantly higher blood concentrations of choline and DHA. These are both essential nutrients for brain development. Another study by the same researchers showed that an egg a day significantly increased growth and reduced stunting by 47% in young children, compared to children who did not eat eggs.

Far too many young children are overweight and many of them will remain overweight throughout their lives, unless changes are made. Sugar-laden snacks and nutrient-poor 'kids' food leave them under-nourished and constantly hungry. A low-carbohydrate diet with plentiful fat and protein from unprocessed, real food can transform these youngsters into healthy, happy and successful people.

Intermittent fasting

Public Health England suggests that we eat 400 calories for breakfast and 600 calories for both lunch and dinner, with 200 calories available for snacks in between. This organisation, along with its counterparts in the rest of the UK, has overseen the obesity crisis without being able to slow it down, never mind reverse it. Dr Jason Fung, a kidney expert in Canada, whom I have mentioned previously, has been able to reduce the weight, and eliminate the symptoms, of his diabetic patients with a different approach. As well as using a low-carbohydrate, high-fat diet, he advocates the use of intermittent fasting. Instead of eating and snacking all day, he has shown that it is much better for our health to spend most of the day not eating. Intermittent fasting is achieved by eating all of our daily food in an eight-hour time period. Eating nothing during the other 16 hours, greatly reduces our insulin levels with considerable metabolic benefits. To achieve this successfully, we need to eat highly nutritious meals of fat and protein that keep us satiated for long periods of time. Dr Fung has proved the benefits of this approach, and it should not be a surprise because it more closely resembles the way we evolved.

Summary,

- Eat real, unprocessed food which comes from a farmer or fisherman and not from a factory.
- Avoid too many carbohydrates, especially sugar, cakes, biscuits, crisps and other 'snacks'.
- Eat plenty of animal-based foods to obtain the nutrients we need. Embrace the flavours and health-giving nourishment of healthy fats and quality proteins.
- Learn to cook, and enjoy, wholesome meals at home with your family and friends.

Chapter 18

ONWARDS TO BETTER HEALTH

Throughout this book I have tried to collate information from an extensive range of sources in my quest to find the truth among all the lies. I have attempted to show that most of the things we have been told about a healthy diet are wrong. We have been misled, and our health has been damaged by egos, religion, politics and money. There are plenty of well-qualified people around the world who are convinced of the benefits of an animal-based, whole food, unprocessed, low-carbohydrate diet. I am just one voice among many. In the immediate future, the vested interests of large organisations will fight back against the facts and logic presented in this book. Eventually the truth will have to be acknowledged but it will take many years for things to change. Whilst newspapers are paid to write anti-livestock stories and scientific journals accept reports that have been paid for by global corporations, the 'experts', who gave us the epidemics of obesity and diabetes, will continue to get the headlines.

The push towards a plant-based diet is gathering momentum and it is backed by what is known as 'Big Food'. This is a collective name for the small group of global corporations that sell processed food to the entire world. They stand to make an even bigger fortune if they persuade us all to give up meat from our local farmers and, instead, eat their ultra-processed, plant-based, laboratory-made fake meat substitutes.

This book explains what has been happening up to now but things will continue to change in the battle for real food. We have been lied to and the lies will continue. I have, therefore, launched a web site, also entitled *Stop Feeding Us Lies*, which will be able to report on, and respond to, everything the purveyors of fake food try to throw at us in the future. The purpose of the site is:

- To respond to new stories, research and advice reported in the media.

- To inform people about the benefits of real food, including animal-based foods, for life-long human health.
- To counteract the malicious propaganda which blames animal agriculture for climate change.
- To help people understand and appreciate the work done by farmers and shepherds.
- To guide and support those people who would like to lose weight by means of a collective weight-loss initiative called *Who wants to lose a Million Pounds?*
- To counteract the constant erosion of our instincts, common sense and freedoms by the ever-growing intrusion into our lives, thoughts, speech and diet by the self-appointed custodians of our lives. These people gave us a long list of modern diseases, a dependency on drugs and the very worst of political correctness. We do not need them.

If you would like to know more about metabolic health and the lies we are told for the benefit of someone else's wealth, please come and join us at:

www.stopfeedinguslies.com

References

Many of my sources of information are quoted in the book. These references, listed by chapter, cover the occasions when I refer to research without a citation.

Chapter 1
1. *Origin, Spread and Demography of the Mycobacterium tuberculosis Complex*
T Wirth et al. Plos Pathology 2008
2. *History of Typhus.* www.medicinenet.com
3. *History of Cholera.* Dhiman Barua
4. *The smallpox story: life and death of an old disease.* Behbehani AM. 1983 *Microbiology Review.*

Chapter 2
1. *Understanding GRADE: an introduction.* Gabrielle Goldet and Jeremy Howick. Department of Primary Health Sciences, University of Oxford
2. *"Saturated fat does not clog the arteries: coronary heart disease is a chronic inflammatory condition, the risk of which can be effectively reduced from healthy lifestyle interventions."* British Journal of Sports Medicine. By Aseem Malhotra, Rita F Redber, Pascal Meier.
3. *Low Fat, Low Cholesterol Diet in Secondary Prevention of Coronary Heart Disease.* Woodhill and Palmer, *Drugs, Lipid Metabolism, and Atherosclerosis*

Chapter 3
1. *Run for your Life.* Noakes T, Spedding M. *Nature*, July 2012
2. Dennis M. Bramble, Daniel E. Lieberman. 'Endurance running and the evolution of Homo'. *Nature*, 2004.
3. *Essential fatty acids and human brain.* Chang CY[1], Ke DS, Chen JY. Department of Neurology, Chi-Mei Medical Center, Tainan Taiwan.

4. *Exercise Induces Hippocampal BDNF through a PGC-1α/FNDC5 Pathway.* C.D/ Wrann et al. *Cell Metabolism* Nov. 2013
5. *Cambridge Encyclopedia of Hunters and Gatherers.* Cambridge University Press. Lee, Richard B.; Daly, Richard Heywood (1999).

Chapter 4

1. *The Biology of Human Starvation.* By Ancel Keys, et al. Univ. of Minn. Press, 1950
2. Lyon, Dunlop (1932) *The treatment of obesity: a comparison of the effects of diet and of thyroid extract.* Quarterly Journal of Medicine
3. *Treatment of obesity: Developments of the past 150 years.* Pennington A. 1954
4. www.epilepsy.org.uk/info/treatment/ketogenic-diet
5. www.diabetes.co.uk/pioneers/william-banting

Chapter 5

1. *Introduction to Lipids and Lipoproteins.* Kenneth Feingold MD. Carl Grunfeld, MD, PhD. www.Endotext.org
2. truemd.com/general-health/the-role-of-cholesterol-in-human-body-metabolism
3. *Lipid regulating drugs.* British National Formulary
4. *Risk of Cognitive Decline Reduced for People 85 and Older With High Cholesterol*
Mountsinai.org March, 2018
5. www.zoeharcombe.com Search 'Rory Collins'
6. www.drmalcomkendrick.org Search 'Rory Collins'
7. www.drmalcolmkendrick.org Cholesterol lowering – proven or not?
8. *Low cholesterol and violent crime.* Golomb BA et al. Journal of Psychiatric Research. Oct 2000

Chapter 6

1. *How much sugar is in your fizzy drink?* Guardian, June 2014
2. *Alzheimer's Disease Is Type 3 Diabetes–Evidence Reviewed.* S de la Monte, J Wands. Journal of Diabetes Science and Technology, Nov. 2008

3. *Prospective Study of Hyperglycemia and Cancer Risk.* P Stattin et al care.diabetesjournals.org Mar 2007

Chapter 7
1. *Possible role of salt intake in the development of essential hypertension. 1960.*
Dahl LK. International Journal of Epidemiology
2. *Sodium intake and mortality in the NHANES II follow-up study.* Cohen et al. American Journal of Medicine. Mar. 2006
3. *Elevated levels of sodium blunt response to stress.* E. Krause et al. The Journal of Neuroscience, Apr. 2011
4. *Exercise-associated hyponatraemia on the Kokoda Track.* D Pattison et al. Medical Journal of Australia, 2011

Chapter 8
1. *Eat Fat, Lose Fat (Chapter 3)* by Dr Mary Enig and Sally Fallon. Penguin Books
2. *Omega-6 vegetable oils as a driver of coronary heart disease.* J. Dinicolantonio & J. O'Keefe. *BMJ Openheart* 2018
3. *Relationship of omega-3 and omega-6 fatty acids with semen characteristics, and anti-oxidant status of seminal plasma: A comparison between fertile and infertile men.* Clinical Nutrition, Feb. 2010

Chapter 9
1. The Global Energy Balance Network ceased to operate at the end of November 2015, after receiving too much negative publicity.
2. *Sugar Industry and Coronary Heart Disease Research* C Kearns et al. JAMA Internal Medicine 2016
3. www.6xc.com.au/lipitor-a-study-in-marketing
4. www.examiner.com.au/story/4094819/board-silences-fettke
5. *The Truth about the Drug Companies: How They Deceive Us and What to Do about It.* Marcia Angell. Random House Books

Chapter 10
1. *Study of Current and Former Vegetarians and Vegans.* Humane Research Council. Dec 2014. faunalytics.org

2. www.diagnosisdiet.com/meat-and-cancer

3. *Health-motivated taxes on red and processed meat: A modelling study on optimal tax levels and associated health impacts.* M Springmann. Plos One. Nov 2018

4. www.openphilanthropy.org/focus/us-policy/farm-animal-welfare/the-guardian-journalism-factory-farming

5. Wikipedia. *Protein poisoning*

6. Frederic Leroy: Health risks of plant-based diets

7. *Micronutrient status and intake in omnivores, vegetarians and vegans in Switzerland.* European Journal of Nutrition. Feb 2017

8. *The Impact of Dietary Organic and Transgenic Soy on the Reproductive System of Female Adult Rat.* American Association for Anatomy. March 2009

9. *Genetically Modified Soy Linked to Sterility, Infant Mortality in Hamsters.* Smith J. Huffpost.com. May 2011

10. Lindeman, Marjaana(2002) 'The state of mind of vegetarians: Psychological well-being or distress?', Ecology of Food and Nutrition

Chapter 11

1. https://dairy.ahdb.org.uk/mycorrhizal-fungi

2. www.fao.org/how-soil-is-destroyed

3. https://oceanservice.noaa.gov/deadzone

4. www.britannica.com/Dust-Bowl

5. *Farmland management changes can boost carbon sequestration rates: Changes can add organic matter to soils much faster than previously thought.* J. Merritt. School of Ecology, University of Georgia

6. www.grasspower.org

Chapter 12

1. *Effects of Exercise Training on Older Patients With Major Depression.* J. Blumenthal et al. Jama Internal Medicine. Oct 1999

2. *Endorphins and Exercise.* Sports Medicine, 1984

3. *The mental and physical health outcomes of green exercise.* International Journal of Environmental Health Research. J Pretty, Oct. 2005

4. *Effects of physical activity on cognitive functioning in middle age*. American Journal of Public health 2005

5. *Poor Physical Performance and Dementia in the Oldest Old*. The 90+ Study. Jama Neurology. Ja. 2013

6. *Effects of exercise on sleep*. S. Youngstedt. Clinics in Sports Medicine. 2005

Chapter 13

1. *Sunshine for your mind*. A. VanHook. Science Signaling. Jul 2018

2. *Here comes the sun to lower your blood pressure*. Science Daily 2014

3. *Vitamin D deficiency during pregnancy tied to autism risk*. Spectrumnews.org

4. *Patterns of COVID-19 Mortality and Vitamin D*. ssrn.com

5. *What is Causing Iran's Spike in MS Cases?* Smithsomian.com

6. *Melanoma is not caused by sunlight*. Christophers AJ. Mutation Research, 1998

7. *Vitamin D_2 Is Much Less Effective than Vitamin D_3 in Humans*. Armas L. Nov 2004 *The Journal of Clinical Endocrinology & Metabolism*

8. *The Link Between a Lack of Sleep and Type 2 Diabetes*. sleepfoundation.org

9. *Sleep, Performance, and Public Safety*. http://healthysleep.med.harvard.edu

Chapter 14.

1. *Children's Aerobic Fitness and Academic Achievement*. American Journal of Public Health 2012. L Cottrel et al.

2. *How does exercise benefit performance on cognitive tests in primary-school pupils?*
Hill & Williams. Developmental medicine and child neurology. Jul 2011

3. *The Relationship of Physical Fitness, Self-Beliefs, and Social Support to the Academic Performance of Middle School Boys and Girls*. The Journal of Early Adolescence. T. Petri. March 2014

4. *Young adults who exercise get higher IQ*. sahlgrenska.gu.se

Chapter 15

1. *So You Think You Know Why Animals Play.* Lynda Sharpe. *Scientific American.* May 2011
2. *Children's Object Manipulation: A Tool for Knowing the External World and for Communicative Development.* V. Focaroli. The Hand.
3. *Consequences of Play Deprivation.* Dr. Stuart L. Brown, National Institute for Play
4. *A world without play.* A review by Play England
5. *Screen-based activities and children and young people's mental health and psychosocial wellbeing: a systematic map of reviews*

Chapter 16

1. *Insulin resistance and outcome in bipolar disorder.* Calkin et al. *British Journal of Psychiatry* Jan 2015
2. *Chronic Schizophrenia Put Into Remission Without Medication.* C Palmer. www.psychologytoday.com April 2019
3. *Catatonia and other psychiatric symptoms with vitamin B12 deficiency.* Berry et al. Acta Psychiatr Scand. 2003
4. *Psychiatric manifestations of vitamin B12 deficiency: a case report.* Durand et al. L'Encephale 2003

Chapter 17

1 *Unprocessed Red Meat and Processed Meat Consumption: Dietary Guideline Recommendations From the Nutritional Recommendations (NutriRECS) Consortium.* Annals of Internal Medicine. Oct 2019
2. *Ascorbic acid: The Forgotten Competition with Glucose.* www.insulean.co.uk
3. *Autism Research 2017: Certain Vitamin, Mineral Deficiencies During Pregnancy May Increase ASD Risk.* Medical Daily June, 2017
4. *The need for animal source foods by Kenyan children.* Bwibo and Neumann. The Journal of Nutrition 2003

Printed in Great Britain
by Amazon